KU-778-111

WITHDRAWN FROM STOCK
DUBLIN CITY PUBLIC LIBRARIES

Hot Dogs & Croissants

Hot Dogs & Croissants

*The Culinary Misadventures of Two French Women
Who Moved to America, Got Fat, Got Skinny (Again),
and Mastered Eating Well in the USA—With Recipes*

Natasha and Victorine Saulnier

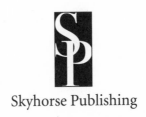

Skyhorse Publishing

Copyright © 2015 by Natasha Saulnier and Victorine Saulnier

All rights reserved. No part of this book may be reproduced in any manner without the express written consent of the publisher, except in the case of brief excerpts in critical reviews or articles. All inquiries should be addressed to Skyhorse Publishing, 307 West 36th Street, 11th Floor, New York, NY 10018.

Skyhorse Publishing books may be purchased in bulk at special discounts for sales promotion, corporate gifts, fund-raising, or educational purposes. Special editions can also be created to specifications. For details, contact the Special Sales Department, Skyhorse Publishing, 307 West 36th Street, 11th Floor, New York, NY 10018 or info@skyhorsepublishing.com.

Skyhorse® and Skyhorse Publishing® are registered trademarks of Skyhorse Publishing, Inc.®, a Delaware corporation.

Visit our website at www.skyhorsepublishing.com.

10 9 8 7 6 5 4 3 2 1

Library of Congress Cataloging-in-Publication Data is available on file.

Cover design by Brian Peterson
Cover photo credit: Thinkstock images

Print ISBN: 978-1-62914-536-5
Ebook ISBN: 978-1-62914-993-6

Printed in the United States of America

Pour Maman et Papa

Table of Contents

Maman's Leek Potato Soup
Serves 4 to 6

- 4 large leeks (Use only the white and pale green parts)
- 3 tablespoons butter
- 5 cups water
- 2 pounds potatoes, peeled, diced into ½ inch pieces
- ¼ cup sour cream
- ¼ cup chopped fresh parsley
- 4 ounces of Swiss cheese
- Salt and freshly ground pepper

1. Cut leeks lengthwise, separate, clean, chop then cook in butter with salt and pepper in a medium sized saucepan.
2. Cover pan, cook on low heat for 15 minutes. Stir leeks once or twice and add a little water if necessary to prevent sticking.
3. Add potatoes and 5 cups water to leeks. Increase heat to medium-high, so that a steady boil can be maintained.
4. Cook about 40–45 minutes, or until the potatoes are tender.
5. Remove from heat.
6. Pulverize potatoes with a handheld blender or transfer the mixture to a blender or food processor and blend until smooth.
7. Mix in salt and freshly ground pepper while soup is still quite hot. Adjust to taste.
8. Top with or mix in parsley.
9. Sour cream and Swiss cheese may be added at any time, if desired.
10. Serve hot.

Chapter One

Hot Dogs or Croissants?

he French countryside flew past the train window as I rummaged inside my handbag searching for sunglasses to hide my red puffy eyes. I had been crying for two days and the pitying looks from my fellow passengers were too much for me to bear. I reached back inside my handbag for a tissue and my hand closed around the letter, that horrible letter. I was tempted to read it again in the vain hope that somehow, stuffed inside its envelope the words had miraculously changed, but what was the use? I knew the devastating news was final. Two years of relentless work reading, analyzing, and deconstructing the greatest works of Chaucer, Nabokov, Hardy, Poe, and too many other authors to name had culminated in nothing but a one-page rejection letter now lying crumpled in my bag. The document informed me that I had failed my *Agrégation d'Anglais*, the civil service exam that would have certified me to teach English literature at a French university. My longtime dream was shattered. All I wanted to do now was run

Leabharlanna Poiblí Chathair Bhaile Átha Cliath
Dublin City Public Libraries

home to my parent's house, curl up in my childhood bed, and disappear. My one consolation? My older sister Victorine would soon be there to share my unhappiness. My mother had informed me during our last tearful phone conversation that Victorine was abandoning London, where she had been living for the last ten years. Nigel, her musician boyfriend, was supplementing his income teaching English as a second language and Victorine had apparently came home unexpectedly early from work and discovered him upstairs in their bed conjugating some irregular verbs with one of his young female Pakistani students. Our father, bravely facing his fear of driving on the "wrong" side of the road, was on a ferry crossing the channel on his way to London in his horse van to retrieve Victorine, her six-toed cat Rani, and her ten years' worth of possessions. No, Spring had not been kind to us Saulnier sisters. We each suffered our own little miseries, mine in Paris, Victorine's in London, and we were both returning to our childhood home in Brittany to lick our wounds.

After three days hiding in my room and replenishing my tears with nothing but hot tea, I finally succumbed to the delicious scents emanating from the pots simmering on my mother's stove. In bathrobe and slippers I shuffled to the kitchen table and sat down to a meal of our favorite childhood dishes. A bowl of Maman's incredible leek potato soup and a large helping of endives covered with béchamel sauce helped to comfort me, and as I finished my first slice of her delicious apple tart my misery began to subside.

"*The world always looks a bit brighter on a full stomach,*" Maman said as she gently stroked my hair and kissed my forehead.

Victorine apparently hadn't lost her appetite, nor skipped a beat, for while I was upstairs sobbing into my pillow, she had been downstairs at the kitchen table drinking coffee, eating crêpes, talking with my parents, reading the brochures she had picked up at the travel agent in town, and most importantly making big plans . . . for the both of us.

As I finished my second slice of apple tart I noticed a spark in her eyes and a look I knew all too well. For as long as I could remember Victorine always kept multiple schemes simmering on the back burners of her mind.

The recent break-up with her now ex-boyfriend had merely turned up the flame under her latest one and it was now boiling over.

"*Natasha,*" she said, "*we're going to America.*"

"*What?*"

"*America,*" she repeated. "*I have it all planned. I explained it all to Maman and Papa and they agree it's a good idea.*"

"*I can't go off on holiday to America now.*"

"*Oh yeah? Why not? What's keeping you here?*" Victorine asked, raising her eyebrows.

I racked my brain for a rational reason why I couldn't go but could find none.

"*Listen, I'm not talking about a holiday, I'm talking about work,*" she continued. "*We'll go back to journalism, like we did before—only this time, we do it in America. I have it all figured out. Contact your editor friend at the newspaper and suggest some story ideas. If he agrees, we'll go.*"

I thought about it. Normally, journalism is a difficult profession to break into in France but through a friend from school who worked at one of France's regional newspapers, I was offered the opportunity to submit a story to the paper's editor several years ago. To my astonishment and delight, he accepted it, then one submission led to the next and the next until eventually, my portfolio had grown to the point that I had the reputation and confidence to submit unsolicited story ideas to editors of a variety of regional newspapers and magazines. Once my proposals were approved, I dove into my research and interviews and wrote stories on topics ranging from politics to culture. Occasionally, Victorine helped me with research and contributed her admirable skills with a camera so I could submit photographs along with the articles.

We hadn't done any reportage while I was engrossed in my studies, but with nothing to keep us in France, Victorine wanted to revive our journalistic selves on the other side of the Atlantic.

"*You have to admit it's a good idea,*" said Victorine as she leaned back in her chair and crossed her arms. "*We both need to get away.*"

She was right, she knew it and she knew that I knew it.

This is how we Saulnier sisters wound up in America, I as a freelance journalist and Victorine as a photojournalist. Like all Europeans, we had heard about the legendary American bonhomie, the relaxed and easygoing attitude of Americans and were eagerly anticipating encountering it firsthand. To be perfectly honest, we were a little tired of some of the French attitudes and the not-so-endearing uptightness and judgmental nature derived from the native sense of superiority. Peek into the psyche of any true French person and you'll find that deep down in their soul, they believe that France is responsible for the invention of all that makes the world civilized: wine, gastronomy, perfume, fashion, and yes, even democracy.

For two romantic and adventurous French girls, America promised to be . . . well, what it is supposed to be, the country of new beginnings and self-reinvention. Like our countryman before us, Alexis de Tocqueville, we wanted to study her mores and customs and learn more about the land we were soon to call the "country of smiles."

Thankfully, language was not an issue. Ten years living in London had left Victorine with an impeccable command of the English language. She had also acquired a noticeably softened accent, both cosmopolitan and elegant, of which I was quite envious. I loathed my strong, unmistakably Parisian accent, but after the umpteenth time I was told it sounded sexy, I decided to embrace it. I had a degree in English Literature after all and aside from the occasional malapropism, felt totally confident in any conversational setting.

Like millions of European immigrants bound for the Free World before us, we landed in New York, and quickly sought out the Statue of Liberty: the famous gift from France symbolizing the friendship between our two countries. The smell of freedom and hope was in the air and the moment we caught sight of her we spontaneously burst out singing the famous Nana Mouskouri song, "Song for Liberty"—a corny song for sure, but we were excited about our newfound freedom. Lady Liberty gazed down upon us impassively. If she knew what was in store for us on our American adventure, she wisely kept it to herself.

Our second day in America was July 4th—Independence Day—and its national festivities were upon us. The newfound New York friends we met on the ferry invited us to Coney Island to give us "Frenchies a real sense of American traditions on Independence Day." Still a bit giddy from the excitement of our arrival in America, we wallowed in the carnival atmosphere and allowed our pals to escort us through crowds that thronged the beachside boardwalk to the Original Nathan's Famous Frankfurters Restaurant. Apparently in America, as in France, national holidays ultimately become all about food, but that's where the resemblance ended. Our joy quickly subsided. We had arrived just in time to catch the starting bell of Nathan's Hot Dog Eating Contest, an annual competition in which each contender's goal is to eat as many hot dogs as possible within the space of twelve minutes. This was something we had never heard about nor could even imagine. We stared dumbfounded at the sight before us: about twenty people standing behind a long table covered with plates piled high with hot dogs and containers of soda. All were frantically stuffing their mouths, sometimes helping themselves with both hands and all ten fingers to broken pieces of hot dogs and buns. The scene was sheer madness. These men and women were gorging themselves non-stop with hot dogs, slurping soda to help them go down, and all the while jumping and squirming like worms in a feeding frenzy. Their faces were red and swollen. The veins on their foreheads and necks protruded. Frankly, they looked as if they were going to vomit. I caught a glimpse of one of the contestants regurgitating some food through his nostrils and I quickly looked away. The screams of hundreds of people attending the contest filled the air. They were rooting for their favorites, yelling their names and egging them on. Just like in a real sports competition, an announcer wearing a straw hat was excitedly pacing the stage and shouting commentary into his microphone.

"Now, only two more minutes to go . . . our champion Joey is considerably slowing the pace . . . Now only fifty-nine seconds to go . . . The crowd is going wilder than ever . . . Now thirty-five seconds to go . . . he's about to set a new world record . . . ten seconds . . . fifty-eight hot dogs! JOEY CHESTNUT IS THE GREATEST EATER IN THE WORLD!"

I was so stunned that I had to borrow a chair from my neighbor, an elderly lady who looked genuinely concerned and kept asking me if I was all right, but the announcer's comments were what really dealt me the final blow.

"I'm truly stunned," he continued, as he stood with the winner at his side. "I've seen some amazing things in my life but this is clearly tops them all, and look at him, he doesn't look affected at all. Isn't it amazing? You've eaten fifty-eight hot dogs and you look healthy and refreshed."

An avalanche of applause and cheers welcomed the announcer's words. To me, the winner didn't look so good at all. A disagreeable situation—and since things can always get worse when you are in a disagreeable situation—an unmistakable smell began to permeate the atmosphere around me. My nose directed my eyes to the guilty parties. Some of the less skilled contestants were doubled over and had begun vomiting in the back. *Great,* I thought, *soon it's going to be my turn.* Yet one question kept turning around my mind: Why on earth would anybody want to hurt oneself so much? I turned to my big sister for an answer. Victorine was sitting motionless, her camera in her lap, staring wide-eyed at the triumphant champion. I got the distinct feeling she was going to throw up, but I was more worried that she might not have taken any photos.

"You didn't take any photos?" I asked.

She didn't answer but instead kept muttering, *"Maman wouldn't like that. Maman wouldn't like that at all."*

Of the two of us, Victorine was the one who at the time had the healthiest relationship with food. She ate no meat, only organic vegetables, and no grease. She lived by the motto, "You are what you eat." Understandably, she was horrified. For French girls who had been taught table manners by an extremely elegant mother, considered by our family on par with any *Cordon Bleu* chef, it was an unimaginable scene, an unfathomable experience. We felt like Martians trapped on an alien planet overrun by a gluttonous species. Our mother had always taught us that quality was more important than quantity in everything, but even more so with food. Didn't the contestants know that they could smother themselves with food? That they were hurting their internal organs? That half of the planet was starving to death?

This inexplicable freak show was our first culinary adventure in the United States—and its morbid and toxic quality left a very bad taste in our mouths. I was never able to write a story about the hot dog eating contest itself. Victorine was so traumatized that she'd only taken three useless photos during the event. Still, we needed to understand what was behind this American tradition. We did some research, and discovered that the truth behind the contest was even scarier than the contest itself.

In 1916, a poor Polish immigrant named Nathan Handwerker made his living slicing bread into buns for ten-cent frankfurters at a restaurant on Coney Island. Nathan's coworkers, Jimmy Durante and Eddie Cantor, singing waiters who would later become famous in their own right, jokingly suggested that Nathan open his own stand and sell them for five cents. Nathan did exactly that. He invested his life's savings of three hundred dollars into his own business on the boardwalk, selling frankfurters made from his wife Ida's own recipe. His slogan: "A hot dog, a pickle, and root beer for a nickel."

Unfortunately, Nathan had a problem. Growing public concern over dubious practices in the meatpacking industry made people doubt the quality of his five-cent hot dogs. At the time, hot dog was a slang term that most likely referred to the fact that the meat from which frankfurters were made was as likely to be dog as anything else.

ECHOS FROM THE LUNCH WAGON
'Tis dogs' delight to bark and bite,
Thus does the adage run.
But I delight to bite the dog
When placed inside a bun.
—From the *Yale Record*, October 5th, 1895

Nathan needed people to trust and believe his hot dogs were healthy. In an inspired, pioneering marketing scheme he hired hungry unemployed actors to don white lab coats, pose as doctors from the nearby hospital, and hang around his stand eating his frankfurters. He then posted a sign reading,

"If doctors eat our hot dogs, you know they're good!" His ploy worked brilliantly. Nathan's Famous quickly became the most popular restaurant on Coney Island and eventually evolved into an American icon. Finally, in 1987, seventy-one years after it first opened with a three hundred dollar investment, Nathan's son Murray sold the family's Nathan's Famous franchise for over nineteen million dollars.

We didn't know it at the time but my sister and I were doomed. We were about to be swallowed by America's fast food culture and our native French way of eating would soon fall completely by the wayside.

Hot dogs or croissants? That was the question. And even as our mother's words rang in our ears—*"Always leave the table a little hungry"*—we would choose hot dogs . . . and we would pay the price.

Murray Handwerker's Cheese Hot Dog Roll-Ups
Serves 4 to 8

- 8 Nathan's Famous Hot Dogs
- 4 slices American cheese
- 1 can crescent refrigerator rolls

1. Preheat the oven 375°F.
2. Parboil hot dogs.
3. Split them lengthwise, almost through.
4. Slice cheese into strips. Insert strips of cheese into each hot dog slit.
5. Separate the crescent rolls into triangles. Wrap each hot dog in a roll.
6. Bake the roll-ups for about 10 minutes or until the rolls turn golden brown.

Source: www.nathansfamous.com

Lotte à l'Américaine
(Monkfish "American Style")
Serves 4

- 2 pounds of monkfish fillets
- 4 tablespoon of olive oil
- 3 big shallots, finely chopped
- 1 small leek, finely chopped
- 3 tablespoons of garlic, finely chopped
- 2 tablespoons of tomato paste
- 1 cup of diced plum tomatoes
- 1 bottle of fruity white wine
- 5 tablespoons of Armagnac or Cognac
- 1 pinch of clove powder
- 1 pinch of grated nutmeg
- Salt and freshly ground pepper
- 1 tablespoon finely chopped parsley

1. Heat the olive oil in a large saucepan until hot.
2. Sauté the garlic, shallots, and leek.
3. Add the tomatoes, tomato paste, salt, pepper, clove powder, nutmeg, white wine, and the Armagnac or Cognac.
4. Let it cook for a few minutes on low medium heat.
5. Add the fillets, cover, and let it simmer gently on low heat for 20 minutes.
6. Sprinkle with parsley and serve hot with rice.

Chapter Two

Deep in the Heart of Texas

We found a small apartment in Astoria, Queens, and spent the next few weeks getting acquainted with New York City's frenetic rhythm, cosmopolitan atmosphere, and multicultural eclectic gastronomy. After a bit of exploration we discovered our neighborhood had a small greengrocer, a decent Portuguese bakery, and a wonderful health food store around the corner where we would stop for a fresh carrot/celery/apple/ginger juice before embarking on our daily excursions. One of our greatest finds while we were settling in was a Middle Eastern restaurant down the street owned by a balding Lebanese man named Sami. On the warm July evenings when it was too hot to go back to our apartment, we sat at one of the tables outside his restaurant, munching triangles of pita bread dipped into plates of hummus and tabouleh salad as Sami repeatedly refilled our glasses of mint tea. We were welcomed customers until one evening when, unexpectedly and unfortunately, Victorine decided to give some unsolicited culinary advice.

"Sami," she said as he passed our table, "your hummus is not bad but I have to tell you, your tabouleh salad . . . Hmm, it's just not right, it's missing something."

Sami stopped cold in his tracks, put his hands on his hips, and turned to look at Victorine suspiciously.

"What?" he began, "You come here every day, you eat my tabouleh. Now you tell me you no like my tabouleh?"

Sensing that Sami didn't appreciate her criticism I quickly shook my head no in answer to his question. He turned, glared at me, and asked,

"Oh, so you no like my tabouleh too, eh?"

"NO . . ." I cried, ". . . I mean yes, I like it . . . I meant no, I don't not . . . like your . . ."

Exasperated, I turned to Victorine, *"Ouf, why did you have to say that? Now he's upset and . . ."*

Victorine ignored me, undeterred and apparently oblivious to the fact she had ruffled any feathers.

"No, it's okay," she said, "but it's missing something . . . you forgot to . . ."

"WHAT? What it's missing?" he asked, then listing the ingredients one by one, with each finger he continued, "I put the couscous, I put the onion, I put the tomatoes, I put the cucumbers, I put the pepper, I put the parsley, I put the mint, I put the olive oil, I put the lemon, I put the salt . . . You tell me what do I not put? . . . eh?"

"You forgot the eggs, the diced hard boiled eggs," replied Victorine.

His body shook as if a sudden jolt of electricity had gone through it then his eyes grew wide and he stared at her incredulously.

"Eggs? . . . EGGS?" he asked, "What kind of idiot puts eggs in tabouleh?"

By this time the heated discussion had caught the attention of the other customers as well as passersby. I braced myself. Sami had unwittingly insulted our Maman, our own personal *Cordon Bleu* chef and I knew Victorine was about to snap.

"Our mother, that's who," she snarled, "and she's no idiot. She knows more about cooking than you could ever hope to in your entire life."

"Fine," he said, noisily stacking our plates and quickly clearing the table, "you go home and have you mother make you food. You French are annoying here just like in Paris. You come my restaurant tell me how to cook . . ."

He continued, muttering to himself and shaking his head as he turned with the tray and disappeared inside.

Victorine jumped to her feet and grabbed her purse.

"Come on, let's get out of here", she huffed.

I sheepishly pulled a ten-dollar bill from my purse and left it on the table as I attempted to invisibly slip from my seat. I caught up to Victorine down the block, waiting at the crosswalk next to a group of people. She was also muttering to herself.

". . . I mean really, it just shows you . . . you try to help someone and there's no appreciation . . . and then, THEN he insults Maman . . ."

"Now, come on," I said, *"He didn't really insult her. Besides, I don't think he needs your advice on how to make tabouleh. It's a dish that came to France from Lebanon after all."*

"Oh, so now you're on his side?" she shrieked, *"He called Maman an idiot. You're going to let him . . ."*

Taking a deep breath, I decided to quit while I was ahead. When Victorine thought she was right, it was pointless to argue. We walked past the shop windows on Astoria Boulevard and I silently nodded yes as Victorine extolled the merits of our mother's cooking and insisted how inferior Sami's food had truly been. That was the last time Victorine ate at Sami's. I returned a few days later by myself, smoothed things over with Sami, and we eventually became friends.

Once we settled in our new neighborhood, America beckoned us and as reporters we were constantly on the go, researching potential stories by day and meeting new interesting people by night. First and foremost, we were eager to get working on the "story of our lives," interviewing two death row inmates in Huntsville, Texas: LaRoyce Smith and Farley Matchett. Years earlier Farley Matchett had been the subject of an exposé in French *Elle* magazine. In our country, where the death penalty has been abolished since 1981 under Mitterrand, he became one of the unwitting faces of the French abolitionist movement. His story captured my imagination and, not without some difficulty, I managed to obtain both Farley and LaRoyce's mailing addresses and had been exchanging letters with them for the past few years. As a true abolitionist, I was convinced they shouldn't be executed. Though I'm not a religious person, I believe that killing another human is wrong and cannot be justified, even if that person is himself a murderer. Of course, I can understand the deeply seated emotional urge of vengeance when a loved one has been killed but I doubt that killing the murderer will bring any true closure to the victim's family. I believe the fact that our society actually "breeds" so many murderers is a very complex problem that has to be tackled intellectually, not emotionally. "Why?" is the question I believe we should be asking ourselves. Preparing for this reportage was turning me into an even more vigorous death penalty opponent. I had requested a meeting with LaRoyce Smith and Farley Matchett through the Texan prison authorities before we left France but so far we had had no response, understandably of course, since Europeans reporters have the reputation of being anti-death penalty and it was reasonable of them to suspect that we weren't coming to visit the death row unit to compliment the guards on the way they handle inmates. When the much-anticipated letter granting us an interview finally arrived, we were overjoyed. I quickly called our newspaper's editor.

"Okay, we'll cover the flight, the rent-a-car, and two days at a motel, but make sure it's a cheap one," he said.

"What? Two days in the Lone Star State isn't enough for us," moaned Victorine after I hung up the phone. "We need at least one week to get acquainted with its people, politics, cuisine, maybe visit a couple of ranches, maybe even J.R. Ewing's! Can you imagine? It's my dream come true. I'm going to meet the descendants of John Wayne, a few country singing cowboys and of course, see some native Indians and American buffalos up close . . ."

Victorine, almost delirious with joy, seemed to be talking to herself more than to me. Her thoughts were now far away, lost in her romantic childhood memories. Those countless evenings spent with our Papa in front of the television watching American western movies; *The Alamo, Stagecoach, Rio Grande, Davy Crockett,* had left an indelible mark on her imagination. That was Victorine's dream, not mine. I couldn't relate as I never fell in cinematic love with any poor lonesome cowboy, I hate guns and I wasn't good on horseback. After a couple of painful falls as a little girl I quickly developed a strong distaste for riding despite our Papa's urging, which, in truth, made it even worse. I wasn't enthused by the thought of riding a fiery purebred and swinging a lasso over my head in the midst of gun toting cowboys. Victorine had always been much more fearless than I. The tomboy of the family, she practically grew up on horseback helping our father with the family business, an equestrian riding club. To be honest, I was considerably more excited about meeting Native Americans who I considered, along with many Europeans, to be wise and spiritual people. Their beautiful nature-oriented names would carry my imagination away to time immemorial when human beings lived close to the earth and took their cues from nature. I can trace my fascination with their culture to when I was young girl reading *Bury My Heart at Wounded Knee* by Dee Brown. Written from the Native American perspective, it carefully documents their displacement and slaughter by the United States government.

We decided to reserve five days for sightseeing in Huntsville before meeting the inmates and the prison officials. The always resourceful and thrifty Victorine had convinced me that since we were on a tight budget, we should use our motel stipend to rent a space in an inexpensive campground and sleep in a tent. As a consolation to me, she made reservations at a campground located near the American Indian reservation of the Alabama-Coushatta tribe of Texas which has occupied approximately 10,000 acres of land in Polk and Tyler counties since the late 1700s, long before Texas became a state.

On what seemed to me the hottest and most humid day in New York City's history, we lugged and loaded our brand new camping gear in and out of subways and shuttle buses to the airport. It was exhausting and by the time we checked our bags and were seated on the plane, my back was hurting, and my blouse was soaked with perspiration from all the crazy exercise. I sighed as I looked worryingly out the window. God, I was dreading those seven nights in Texas, trying to sleep in a tent on the hard ground. Unlike Victorine, who can sleep like a log anytime, anywhere, I tend to have insomnia when I'm stressed. I kept thinking about the letters of LaRoyce and Farley and their vivid descriptions of the death row unit where they were locked up. As our plane left the runway and climbed into the sky I looked over at Victorine. She was wearing her sunglasses and happily tapping her feet while singing along with the country music blaring on her headset.

We landed in Houston and the suffocating heat almost knocked me down when I stepped out of the air-conditioned airport; but the adventure and the road trip were beckoning us and my heart was pounding. We picked up our bulky baggage, wheeled it over to pick up our rental car and were surprised to find we had been upgraded to a red sedan, two sizes up from the economy one we had reserved.

"*That's a sign, Natasha*. Thank you Texas!" Victorine sang triumphantly.

The unspoken designated driver, Victorine checked the map, plotted a course from Houston to Livingstone which avoided highways and made a detour through Sam Houston National Forest. The drive in the countryside was relaxing and the warm sun and breeze on my face calmed me as I watched lush green pastures and tall green trees slip past my passenger window. She was driving very cautiously, maybe a little too slowly for the wide Texan roads.

"*Double entendre*," she said, pointing to the third "DON'T MESS WITH TEXAS" sign we saw on the side of the road. "*Obviously, they don't just mean keep the place clean. They mean don't get caught doing something bad here, or you might end up in jail for life.*"

Two hours later we arrived at the Coushatta Family Campground in Livingston. It was a large green field scattered with shade trees set in the middle of a thick forest. Trailers, tents, and mobile homes were lined up in neat little rows extending out from a central community bathroom and shower facility. Children wearing bathing suits and riding bicycles chased each other around the dusty dirt road circling the park. A man tended his barbecue grill outside his trailer while a young woman in cut off jean shorts and bikini top hung towels to dry on a clothesline strung up on her camper's awning. At the registration office we found the owner, a friendly pot-bellied, bald man who insisted we call him "Big Jim."

"Okay ladies, I have your reservation right here," he said, "Seven nights for Natasha and Vick-to . . . Vick-tor . . ."

"Victorine," I said, helping him with the pronunciation, "It rhymes with Tangerine."

"Vick-tor-een, Vick-tor-een," he repeated, "Well, that's a new one on me. Vick-tor-een and Natasha, two very pretty names for two very pretty ladies . . . if you don't mind me sayin'. Well, I have a nice campsite picked out for ya. It's over by the edge of the field, close to the trees, so you'll have some privacy, but not too far from the showers."

"Thank you very much, Jim," said Victorine.

"Big Jim, call me Big Jim," he bellowed with a laugh, "Happy to oblige. Just let me know if you need anything, anything at all."

"Well actually there is . . . Big Jim," I said, "I understand we are close to the reservation of the Alabama-Coushatta. Do you know how we could meet with some members of the tribe?"

"You want to meet some Indians?" he said with a laugh, "Well shoot, that's easy. You take a right out of the driveway and head down the road right there a piece to the first fillin' station. Right next to it you'll see a market. If you head over there right 'bout now there's a good chance you'll see three old-timers sittin' outside." He glanced at his wristwatch. "Yup, those three are always just sittin' out there this time of day."

Big Jim was right. Outside the market in the shade of an awning sat three men in a row on plastic patio chairs, watching us as we drove into the parking lot. All three were dressed in jeans, white T-shirts, and baseball caps. Each held a bottle of Coca-Cola. From their handsome features and darker complexion they were easily recognizable as Native American. We stepped out of the car and Victorine walked resolutely towards them. I trailed along, a few steps behind, both enraptured and intimidated. I had no idea how to strike up a conversation with these men but starting conversations was never a problem for Victorine.

"Do you belong to the Alabama-Coushatta tribe?" she asked the three of them.

All three of them studied her for a moment then one of them answered, "Yes," and the other two just nodded.

Their faces were wrinkled like old prunes and their statue-like stares betrayed no emotion as they calmly sat and watched us with their dark eyes. A pickup truck entered the parking lot, pulled up in front of the market, and two skinny cowboys in tight jeans and cowboy hats and boots climbed out of the cab. As they walked toward the entrance they noticed Victorine talking to the three men and eyed us both suspiciously. Victorine didn't notice. She was on a mission.

"We're reporters from France doing a story in Huntsville. My name is Victorine and this is my little sister Natasha," she said glancing back in my direction. "My little sister is a bit shy," she added. I rolled my eyes in irritation.

"Nice to meet you. My name is Clayton," the youngest looking of the three answered, "These are my friends Clem and Roland."

Victorine flashed her sweetest smile and continued excitedly.

"It's really an honor for us to meet you today. When we were little girls, we really enjoyed watching American western movies with our father."

The three men sat up a bit straighter, their eyes narrowed slightly and they continued staring at us.

"*Hey, those weren't my favorite memories,*" I said to Victorine in French, "*and didn't you stop to think that maybe they weren't the fondest ones for them either. Let me do the talking before you make a bigger fool of yourself.*"

"You'll have to excuse my sister, Clayton," I said, "She's a little excited to meet you because we Europeans have a huge admiration for Native Americans. We believe they belong to the few wise societies left on the planet who still live in harmony with Mother Earth."

I guessed I had said the right thing because the three men looked at each other then back to us and smiled broadly.

"Do you mind if I ask you a little bit about your history?" I asked.

"No, go right ahead," answered Clayton, "What would you like to know?"

"I understand your tribe is called the Alabama-Coushatta but you're here in Texas. Is there a story behind that name?" I asked.

"Yes, our tribe originally lived in the area that is now Mississippi and Alabama but we were pushed here in the late eighteenth and early nineteenth centuries by the European-American settlers. In nineteen eighty-seven, we were officially recognized as the Alabama-Coushatta Tribe of Texas," Clayton explained.

"How many people are there in your tribe?" I asked.

"About eleven hundred people who live on about forty-five hundred acres of reservation," said Roland.

The men were friendly but reserved. Their facial expression and tone of voice were in tune with the legendary wisdom I had imagined. Clayton turned to look at his two friends for a moment then turned back to us.

"Would you like to join us at our home for dinner this evening?" Clayton asked, "We have a special catch from the lake today."

We looked at each other, smiled and nodded yes enthusiastically. All we had eaten for lunch was a bag of potato chips and pretzels that we picked up at a gas station on the drive from the airport. I grabbed my notebook from the car and Roland drew a small map to help us navigate our way inside the reservation.

"Come at sunset," he said.

Our mouths were already watering as we rushed back to the campground to shower and change for dinner. We wondered aloud what sort of wonderful freshwater creature our stomachs would have the privilege of digesting that evening. Perhaps it would be a shimmering rainbow trout, a big whiskered catfish or a largemouth bass? What kind of delicious Native American sauce filled with indigenous herbs would the fish be simmering in? Being natives of the Breton seashore, we both loved seafood.

"Mmm, right now I'd like to be sitting down to a plate of Maman's Lotte à l'American," said Victorine smacking her lips, *"do you remember how she prepares it?"*

She was referring to one of our mother's signature dishes, Monkfish with a tomato and white wine sauce, "American style," Monkfish, with its flat head and huge scary mouth is one of the ugliest fishes in the market but it tastes delicately divine and its firm flesh stands up to strong flavorful sauces.

"Of course I remember," I answered, *"She braises the fish in olive oil, onions, garlic, parsley, tarragon, tomatoes, and white wine."*

I closed my eyes and memories of the aroma of that unbelievable sauce simmering on the stovetop and filling the entire house came back to me.

"Yes," said Victorine, *"but I know Maman's secret. First she browns the fish slightly then covers it with Armagnac."*

I opened my eyes, turned to look at Victorine and we yummed in unison, like a couple of hungry stray cats.

"Yes, I remember," I sighed, *"Thinking about it now is making me happy and homesick at the same time."*

We arrived at the reservation just after sunset, our French taste buds were going crazy anticipating a real meal lovingly prepared by incredible cooks. As we entered the gates, I began laughing but quickly caught myself.

"What's so funny?" asked Victorine.

"Oh, nothing," I answered.

"Tell me," she insisted.

"Well . . . I realized that I'd been subconsciously expecting . . . hoping to walk into a tipi village filled with Indians sporting full regalia; breechcloths, leggings, shawls, headdresses, beaded moccasins," I admitted sheepishly.

She rolled her eyes.

"Oh, and an eagle feather war bonnet or two I suppose," she chided, *"Don't be ridiculous."*

I knew she secretly wished the same thing. What we did find was a group of about twenty to twenty-five people preparing a lovely outdoor picnic in the yard outside a cluster of one-story white clapboard houses nestled in a glade of pine trees. Women were setting buffet platters on a long outdoor table, children were playing ball nearby, and the men were seated around an open campfire pit. Our three new friends waved to us as we approached and Clayton motioned to us to join him by the campfire. We made the round of introductions, then each person went back to their dinner preparations. We were simply mesmerized by the huge cooking pot hanging over the fire. The scents of shallots, aromatic herbs, and potatoes reaching our nostrils confirmed what we already knew: it was going to be delicious. Roland sat next to us smiling.

"So, what is cooking in the mysterious pot? It smells absolutely delicious," I asked curiously.

"It's a turtle soup," Roland answered in a matter-of-fact tone.

I thought I had misheard him. Victorine didn't quite get it either. "A what?" she asked.

"Snapping turtle soup. It is a delicacy for our tribe."

I continued staring at the pot but somehow it didn't register. Did he mean a mock turtle soup as in *Alice in Wonderland*?

Victorine cleared her throat. As usual, in a delicate situation, she kept her cool better then I.

"Oh . . . Do you actually mean that there is a real snapping turtle in that pot?" she asked, maintaining a calm straight face. I admired her more than ever because I was repulsed at the thought of eating a snapping turtle and had difficulty removing the disgusted look from mine. Clayton and Roland both nodded and pointed to an enormous gnarled and spiked brown oval shell the size of a large serving platter leaning against a large rock next to the campfire. I instantly lost my appetite and was about to apologize, pretend I was sick, and say I needed to return precipitously to the campground when Victorine caught my nauseated grimace and flashed me a severe look. I realized I'd better sit still so I tried to look pleased and just listened to Roland.

"My son and I caught this snapping turtle in the lake this morning. He was big, about forty pounds so believe me, he was a tough one to land. He snapped at us a few times and then, when we put him on the chopping block he pulled its head and feet under its shell. We waited for him to calm down, then when he stuck his head out again I waved a broom handle in front of his nose. He grabbed onto that good and hard with his jaws and I pulled and pulled. Just when I had his head pulled out nice and far, WHAM, my son cut off his head with the axe in one slice and . . ."

I let out an uncontrolled shriek and at once all eyes turned towards me. Roland's voice stopped suddenly as he noticed the look of horror on my face. Maybe my complexion didn't look so good either. I was trying as hard as I could not to imagine the poor turtle's agony but I kept envisioning his legs flailing and his bleeding disembodied head floating in the soup. The urge to leave was getting stronger and stronger.

"Are you alright?" asked Clayton

"Yes, I'm fine," I answered, "I'm sorry for screaming like that but Roland's story took me by surprise."

"I'm sorry," said Roland, "I didn't mean to scare you."

"No, that's alright," I answered, "I was just thinking about that poor turtle suffering like . . ."

"I don't believe he suffered," interrupted Clayton, "He fought bravely right up to the end and he died quickly and cleanly. Roland and his son made sure of that."

"Oh, I didn't mean that they . . ." I began to apologize but Clayton wasn't finished.

" . . . That old boy has been living in that lake for many, many years," he continued. "Judging by his size and strength I'd say he had a good long life and was probably older than both of you. He was a hunter himself and most likely had many offspring who will take his place. Today was his day to pass."

I looked around and saw Roland and the other men staring into the fire, nodding silently in agreement. My eyes settled upon Victorine who was watching Clayton and Roland intently.

"I think I understand," she said, "You sound as if you have, well, had respect for him."

"Yes of course," said Roland smiling as he looked to Victorine, "I have respect for his spirit. We showed our respect for him in the way that we took his life—quickly and cleanly. When he grabbed hold of that broom handle he was fighting bravely, not cowering or scared. My son made certain the axe blade was very sharp so he could slice off his head with one blow."

I caught myself wincing when I heard this again. Victorine saw it and shot me a reproving look.

"You see, he lived his life according to his true nature," said Clayton, "He was able to live free as a turtle and all living creatures should. Now, consider this: not far from here are factory farms where they raise chickens that are hatched, live, and die in huge windowless coops, never seeing the sun their entire short lives. To me, that's cruelty."

"You're right," said Victorine, "The treatment of animals in those factory farms is inhumane."

"Not only that," continued Clayton, "When you eat the flesh of an animal that has been mistreated like that, you are taking that pain and suffering and making it a part of yourself."

As I listened to Clayton speak I looked up at the faint stars appearing in the darkening evening sky. His soothing voice had a calming effect. I felt the warmth of the fire on my face and thoughts swirled in my head. The smell of the wood smoke brought me back to my childhood summer evenings on my grandparent's farm in Brittany, near the sea in the northwest corner of France. Although small, the farm was our wonderland where we spent our summer vacations with horses, apples trees, goats, a vegetable garden, and a flock of chickens who ran around the farm freely and laid eggs for us to make a game of searching for each morning. It was a far cry from our home in the congested Paris suburbs where we lived at that time. My thoughts went to Louis, my grandmother's grey goose that strutted around the barnyard as if he was the king of the farm when suddenly Clayton's words brought back a memory, a memory I had tucked away and didn't want to think about.

One summer when I was very, very young, our grandfather, a horse breeder and trader, brought Victorine and me with him on a long road trip to deliver a prize Arabian mare to a farm northeast of Bordeaux in the beautiful lush green region called Périgord, in the Dordogne. Once at the farm, while our grandfather unloaded the horse and attended to business with its new owner, Victorine and I, hand in hand, went off to explore and look at the farm animals. Drawn by the sound of geese honking we wandered into a large barn and were surprised to find it filled with rows and rows of geese, hundreds of them, each in a tiny cage with its neck sticking out the top. Wide eyed and scared we stood frozen as we watched as a man went from one bird to the next, grabbing it by the neck and forcing down its throat a long tube attached to what looked like a giant vacuum cleaner. He held the tube down each bird's throat for a moment, pulled it out and held its beak closed as the bird, obviously in pain, struggled and fought to free itself. Horrified, I let go of Victorine's hand and ran out of the barn crying and yelling, *"Louis, Louis he's hurting Louis."* All I could think of was our beloved grey goose Louis being tortured that way. I was inconsolable until we arrived back at our grandparent's farm. I ran to find Louis, hugged him, and assured him no one would ever hurt him that way. Victorine and I later learned that we had unwittingly stumbled upon what is called *"le gavage,"* the practice of forced over-feeding of geese and ducks in order to induce the disease Hepatic Steatosis, which causes their livers to grow to as much as ten times their normal size. This is done in order to produce the famous French delicacy *"foie gras"* or to be exact, fatty liver. I was jolted back from my memories by the sound of Victorine's voice.

"Yes, I would love to try some of your soup," Victorine said politely, "and I'm sure Natasha would love to try it also," she added in a louder voice as she glared at me. I was about to decline when Clayton placed a steaming bowl in my hands. His sweet demeanor calmed me and I knew I would insult our hosts if I refused. Besides, everyone was scrutinizing my expression. I looked down at the murky soup. It was ominously dark with little cubes of meat. The meat looked a little bit like pork with soya sauce but strangely enough, it smelled delicious. I looked at Victorine. She was breathing deeply, stoically bringing a full spoon to her mouth.

"I've never tried turtle but you know, in our country, we eat snails and frogs' legs," she said with a laugh. Then, slurp; she swallowed a spoonful of soup. My eyes opened wide.

"It's really delicious," she said, smacking her lips.

Everybody was smiling, then all the eyes turned to me and I knew the time had come for my own brave deed. So, I followed in my older sister's footsteps and slowly brought the spoon to my mouth. I hesitated a moment, inhaled the . . . well . . . attractive scent, then took a sip of the warm liquid. Miraculously, it tasted delicious, like a very aromatic mix of chicken, pork, and veal. I smiled victoriously. Victorine nodded in approval then voraciously finished her bowl. I could tell from the look in her eyes that she was about to ask for more.

Our soup was just the first course of a lovely meal of homemade dishes prepared from the gardens of our gracious hosts. Sitting at the long table, surrounded by Clayton and Roland's large family, I was again reminded of our grandparent's farm and our evening meals seated at their outdoor table in the garden. I thought of the words our grandmother, quoting Jean Anthelme Brillat-Savarin, the famous French writer and gastronome, would say, *"Tell me what you eat and I will tell you what you are."* This saying was epitomized in our two hosts, Clayton and Roland. Their wisdom reminded us that we are part of a large circular food chain and kindness and compassion for all living things is the key to our healthy survival.

Clayton's Snapping Turtle Soup

- 1 pound Snapping Turtle meat, cubed
- 1 tablespoon of butter
- ¼ cup garlic, minced
- 1 onion, chopped
- 4 celery, chopped
- 4 potatoes, quartered
- 4 carrots, quartered
- 1 gallon of beef stock
- 1 sprig of rosemary
- 1 sprig of thyme
- 2 bay leaves
- 1 tablespoon of cayenne pepper

1. In a large soup pot add butter and sauté the garlic, onion, and the celery until soft.
2. Add the turtle meat and cook until nearly tender.
3. Add the gallon of beef stock with the potatoes, carrots, rosemary, thyme, bay leaves, and the cayenne pepper. Let it simmer covered for 1 hour.

Crêpes Sarrasin au Jambon et Fromage
(Buckwheat Crêpes with Ham and Cheese)
Makes approximately 12 crêpes

- 2 eggs
- 1 cup of buckwheat flour
- 1 cup of whole milk
- 1 cup of water
- 2 cups of Swiss cheese
- 12 slices of ham
- 4 tablespoons of melted butter
- Salt and pepper

1. Combine the flour and salt in a bowl.
2. Form a well in the center of the bowl. Pour in the egg mixture and the cup of water.
3. Mix the batter with a blender or handheld mixer and at the same time pour slowly the cup of milk and the butter. Continue mixing for about 3–4 minutes until the batter is smooth.
4. Let the crêpe batter rest for at least 2–3 hours.
5. Place your frying pan over medium heat. Grease it with a knob of butter.
6. Pour about ½ cup of the batter in the center of the pan. Lift the pan and then tilt and rotate it until the batter is evenly spread. Lower the heat to low.
7. Flip crêpe once then place a slice of ham and sprinkle some cheese on top. Let the cheese melt for a couple of minutes. Fold the crêpe in on all 4 sides leaving the filling exposed.
8. Repeat until the batter is gone.

Chapter Three

French Heifers at the Watering Hole

O ddly enough, my night's sleep was very restful. Maybe it was my full stomach and the wonderful evening of conviviality with real gentlemen. At seven a.m. we unzipped the tent flap and were met by a glorious smiling sun and birds singing a cheerful welcome to the day.

"First, let's have a good Texan breakfast and then I want to explore some back roads and see some of the countryside," said Victorine cheerfully.

"Great idea," I said.

The warmth of the early morning sun suggested it was going to be a blazing day. Ten minutes down the road we found a little place called the Armadillo Diner with a line of dusty pickup trucks parked outside. With its flat roof, faded wooden siding and rectangular shape, it looked straight out of an old western movie. That was enough to trigger Victorine's Wild West imagination.

"Just imagine a saloon right there with swinging doors, beautiful women singing and dancing inside, gunfights at night, horses tied up outside. Can you hear a harmonica and a tinny piano playing that old fashioned music?"

She whistled the haunting theme from "The Good, the Bad and the Ugly." *"Don't you get the chills?"* she asked, bouncing with excitement.

I laughed. Her exhilaration was contagious, or maybe I was just starting to enjoy Texas. I joined her reverie and could almost hear our spurs jingling as we entered and crossed to the counter like a couple of hungry cowboys fresh off the trail. The breakfast patrons looked up from their plates and scrutinized us as we walked by. The waitress, a plump peroxide blonde wearing a skimpy skirt and a tight white T-shirt, turned and greeted us with a wide grin as we sat down.

"Howdy! Y'all want some coffee?"

"Yes, coffee and we would like a Texan breakfast," said Victorine.

"Yup, a cowgirl breakfast," I said, giggling at my own silliness.

"Ah, y'all aren't from 'round these parts are ya?" she asked as she wrote down our order.

"No, we're from Paris but we currently live in New York," Victorine answered.

"I've got a cousin who lives in Paris . . . Paris, TEXAS!" she snorted, laughing loudly at her own joke, probably not for the first time.

"All rightly, two Dale Evans skillets comin' right up," she said, still chuckling to herself as she turned and left to put in our order.

She returned with a steaming pot of coffee and filled our mugs.

"So, how do you gals like Texas?"

She was the bubbly, friendly type. I was trying to think quickly how to answer this difficult question.

"Well, very different for sure . . ." I started to answer but Victorine jumped in. She was in a playful mood.

"For starters, we don't have any cowboys back at home . . . which is a real shame," she said, then turned to look directly at two handsome blue-eyed cowboys who were sitting at the far end of the counter staring at us. They politely lifted their hats in unison as one of them said, "Howdy ladies."

Victorine flashed one of her biggest smiles and answered with a musical, *"Bonjour."*

I could feel my face turn bright red. I gave her thigh a hard pinch under the counter and hissed under my breath, *"What are you doing? Stop!"*

The waitress burst out laughing but was interrupted by the cook glaring at her through the service window and furiously ringing the order bell.

Victorine ignored me, stared straight ahead, and sipped her coffee with a mischievous smile. I leaned forward and snuck a peek at the two cowboys who were now hunched over their plates, speaking quietly beneath the wide brims of their hats while sneaking discreet glances at the two of us.

Our waitress returned with two huge plates loaded with food: two fried eggs, sausage, bacon, biscuits covered with gravy, and a small bowl filled with a whitish substance I didn't recognize topped with a square of melting butter.

"Oh my god, it's enormous," I involuntarily exclaimed.

"I'll be right back with your orange juices. It comes with your orders," the waitress said.

"I guess everything is bigger in Texas. Your eyes are bigger than your stomach," Victorine said, quoting our mother, as she always did when the subject was food. She was right. Like most French women, our breakfast is usually light, just a bowl of *café au lait* (coffee with milk) and fresh bread or a croissant or perhaps a crêpe with a little butter or jam, something to tide us over till midday when we normally have our most substantial meal. I looked down at the plate in front of me and thought maybe I wasn't cut out to be a cowgirl after all.

"We're certainly not going to go hungry while we're here," I said. I had no idea how prophetic my statement would turn out to be. I looked over at Victorine who was finishing the last spoonful of the white butter-topped substance I couldn't identify just as the waitress was returning with our juices.

"Yum, what is this?" Victorine asked the waitress.

"That's grits. Why honey, you never had grits?" the waitress replied with true disbelief in her voice.

"No, what are they?" she asked, snatching the bowl from my plate and gobbling up mine before I could say a word.

"It's just cornmeal," she said, "boiled up with a little salt . . ." then after a quick glance over her shoulder towards the kitchen she leaned closer and continued in a conspiratorial whisper, " . . . well, that's how Frank makes 'em here but let me tell you, you ain't tasted nothin' till you tried my grits. I call 'em cheesy grits."

"Cheesy grits?" Victorine repeated, her eyes growing wide.

"Yup," she answered, "They're super easy to make but nothin' tastes better. I'll tell you how to make 'em. First off, go to the store and get yourself a package of . . . hominy grits."

She pulled out the pen tucked behind her ear, tore a page from her order book and began to write.

"Now, don't go buyin' instant grits. Get yourself regular grits and if you can, make sure the package says stone ground."

Victorine nodded and repeated, "Stone ground hominy grits."

"That's right," our waitress said, nodding as she continued writing, "you'll taste the difference right away. Now, what you do is add a little salt to three cups of water and bring it to a boil. Once it's boilin', slowly stir in about one cup of grits and keep stirrin' till they start boilin' again, then you turn down the heat and let them simmer for about twenty minutes. Keep an eye on them so they don't burn and stir them often, you don't want them to get lumpy."

Victorine nodded again.

"Once they're cooked and lookin' nice and creamy you stir in some black pepper, one or two tablespoons of butter and about one half cup of grated cheese. I like to use sharp cheddar. Just stir everything in till the cheese is melted."

"Yum, cheesy grits," Victorine repeated licking her lips.

"Yup," said our waitress handing Victorine the paper with her recipe and name, Mona written on the bottom.

"You'll be spoiled for anything else and it's the perfect breakfast when you have a hangover." She began to laugh but was interrupted again by the ringing of the cook's order bell.

The two cowboys, one with dark hair and chiseled features, the other with blond hair and a typical American square jaw tipped their hats goodbye as they passed us on the way out the door. I smiled as I watched them leave.

"*Two distinguished cowboys, who would have thought?*" I said wistfully, "*Maybe I am going to like Texas, after all.*"

"*What, what are you talking about?*" said Victorine.

"*They're gone,*" I said, "*Your cowboys just walked out.*"

"*Oh,*" She said barely looking up. She hadn't noticed. She was enraptured by her newfound love . . . grits.

Neither of us touched the sausage or bacon but the eggs and warm biscuits were delicious and the coffee was strong. We finished our breakfast, paid our bill, thanked Mona and left, ready to tour the countryside. We stepped out the front door into the bright sun and immediately stopped in our tracks, taken by surprise. The two cowboys were directly outside, casually leaning against a large pickup truck, their hats tilted back on their heads and their eyes hidden by dark sunglasses.

"Hello again ladies, y'all ain't from 'round here, are ya?" the blond asked.

"No, we're from France," Victorine answered with her most engaging smile, as she raised her hand to shade her eyes from the sun.

"From France? Well, you two sure are a long way from home. What are you doing way out here?" the dark-haired one asked.

"Oh, we're just doing a little sightseeing," answered Victorine.

"Well, pleased to meet you," he said, "This is Jack and my name's Lynn."

"I'm Victorine and this is my little sister Natasha."

I must remember to tell her to drop the "little" once and for all, I thought.

He looked at both of us over the top of his sunglasses and continued, "Well, since you're sight-seeing, maybe Jack and I can show you a few local sights," he said with a wide grin.

I nodded yes enthusiastically but still couldn't seem to find my voice.

"Oh, we wouldn't want you to go to any trouble just for us," said Victorine.

"It would be our pleasure, ladies," said Jack, the one with blond hair.

"Well then, yes, that would be very nice of you," said Victorine, managing to maintain an air of friendly nonchalance. "We would love to see some of the real Wild West, a rodeo or maybe a ghosty town."

Jack let out an involuntary laugh then quickly collected himself. Lynn looked back at Jack whose head was now lowered, trying to hide his amusement behind the wide brim of his hat. Lynn turned back to us smiling.

"Well, I don't know about any . . . ghosty towns round these parts," he said, turning again to look at Jack who had let out another little laugh, "but we could sure take you to the rodeo. Tell you what ladies. Jack and I have some business we have to take care of back at the ranch. How about we meet you later, right here at say, eight o'clock. Is that good for you?" he asked as he removed his sunglasses and looked straight into my eyes.

I felt my face flush then quickly nodded yes and looked to Victorine for help.

"Yes, that sounds fine," she said.

Jack and Lynn climbed in their pickup, and as they drove out of the parking lot Victorine turned to me and said, *"What's wrong with you? You didn't say a word, not even hello or goodbye! Come on, let's go."*

We got in our car and headed towards a park Victorine had found on the map. It had a lake where we could swim. We drove for a while in silence. She was right. I've never been at a loss for words but this handsome Texan had an effect on me that was a bit disconcerting, and I liked it. I was glad that Victorine chose not to bring up the fact that we were journalists, here to do a story on death row inmates. At that moment I wasn't in the mood to have a contentious conversation with our two handsome cowboys. The bright sun was warming my face, and I had a sense of peacefulness mixed with underlying excitement. Right then, just as Lynn had said, I felt very far from home. Victorine interrupted my thoughts.

"Wait a minute, did he say they had something to take care of back at the RANCH?"

"Yes, I think so," I said, after thinking for a moment.

"Maybe they're real cowboys!" she said, and we both laughed.

I turned on the car's radio and searched up and down the dial.

"I can't find anything but country music and evangelical preachers," I moaned.

"Well, if we're going to be hanging around cowboys, I'd advise we stick to country music," said Victorine.

There was no countering such a persuasive line of reasoning. Johnny Cash and Willie Nelson were of course my favorites but I quickly developed a taste for more modern singers like George Strait, Keith Urban, Tim McGraw, Brad Paisley, Kenny Chesney, Toby Keith, and Hank Williams Jr. By the late afternoon, after driving around the countryside, taking a dip in a nearby lake, and smiling back and replying "howdy" to close to a dozen genial locals, I was turning into a country music fan and my chilly attitude toward Texas and Texans was thawing.

Back at the campground we prepared for our evening's rendezvous. From the bottom of our backpacks, Victorine and I pulled out the discreet knee-length dresses we had packed for just such an unexpected night out. Mine was beige, Victorine's red. With flat leather sandals, very little makeup and our hair down we looked casually elegant, the French way. We had no idea what the evening had in store for us but it was Friday night and yes, we had come to Texas for work but after all, one lives only once.

We purposely arrived at the Armadillo Diner a few minutes fashionably late and found our two handsome cowboys slouched against their pickup truck. They recognized our car as we entered the parking lot and stepped forward to greet us. In the soft glow of the setting sun with their black Stetson hats, crisp black shirts, blue jeans, and boots they looked dashing. I had promised myself I wouldn't be tongue tied as I was this morning but Lynn's deep blue eyes caught mine as he approached and my resolve weakened. What was wrong with me? They both removed their hats as we stepped out of the car.

"Good evening ladies," said Lynn.

"Yes, good evening ladies," said Jack, "We weren't sure you'd come."

"Well of course we came," I said, surprising myself with my response. "You said you'd show us some sights, so here we are. Where are we going?"

"To the rodeo of course, that's where you said wanted to go right?" said Jack with a sly smile.

"Now? We're going to the rodeo now?" I asked in dismay. "But, we're not dressed for . . ."

"Yes, yes, yes. Let me get my camera," cried Victorine excitedly as she turned to run back to our car.

Lynn and Jack both laughed.

"Hold on ladies, Jack's just playin' with you," said Lynn. "We thought we would take you to a little place called Midnight Rodeo. It's a dance hall, a saloon where we can have a few drinks and do some dancing. Would you like that?" Lynn asked, looking into my eyes and smiling.

"What a marvelous idea" I replied, entranced by Lynn's beautiful deep blue eyes but a bit skeptical about my dancing abilities.

Surprisingly, they hadn't paid us any compliments on our appearance or outfits, which was the typical behavior of a French man. How disappointing for we had paid extra attention to our looks and tried to dress nicely. I wondered if our efforts had gone unnoticed or if this was a typical Texan trait. The four of us climbed into the huge front cab of their pickup truck and we drove off to start our evening.

Lynn pulled off the highway and parked in front of a huge building covered with blinking lights and neon sign atop which read "Midnight Rodeo." Dozens of cars and pickups crowded the huge parking lot and a parade of would be cowboys and cowgirls were swarming toward the front entrance. As I stepped out of the truck I could hear an upbeat country tune I recognized from the car radio this afternoon thumping loudly inside. We joined the crowd pushing toward the entrance. A huge cowboy, arms folded, standing like a sentry looked Victorine and me up and down as we approached. He then looked over at our escorts and his face broke into a wide grin.

"Why, howdy fellers, evening ladies," he said tipping his hat.

He gave them a wink, shook their hands, and laughed when Jack leaned in to say something I couldn't make out over the din of the music.

"A friend of yours?" I asked as we stepped inside.

"Yes, that's Luke. He's a rodeo clown and a bouncer when he's not out on the circuit," said Lynn. "Can we get you ladies a beer?"

We both nodded yes and I was about to ask what he meant by "rodeo clown" but my attention was immediately drawn to the scene in front of me. The inside of Midnight Rodeo was enormous. Dominating the center of the room was a large rectangular bar surrounded by a layer of people three deep, waving cash, vying for the attention of the harried bartenders who were serving bottles of beer and pouring drinks. A sea of cowboy hats stretched in front of me as far as I could see through the smoky haze. To our right was a line of about a dozen pool tables with players hunched over them, carefully lining up their shots. Behind them, against the wall was a long line of pinball machines, all flashing and ringing as players furiously pounded their buttons. To the left was a giant tennis court sized dance floor, filled with rows and rows of line dancers, all facing the same direction, jumping and stepping in unison to the loud country beat. Victorine was next to me jumping up and down, smiling and clapping.

"*I feel like we stepped into 'Urban Cowboy,'*" I said to her.

"*I wonder if our cowboys dance as well as John Travolta,*" she said, looking over her shoulder at Lynn and Jack who were returning from the bar with a round of beers.

We immediately noticed our dresses looked quite plain compared to the flashy outfits of the women. Skimpy tees showing off as much cleavage as possible on top and skintight boot-cut jeans or miniskirts with the ubiquitous cowboy boots. (We later heard to our dismay that the most coveted pairs of boots were made from alligator, eel, and ostrich). The men were all wearing the same uniform of snug-fitting jeans, crisp western shirt, cowboy hat, boots, and a wide belt with a big silver buckle adorned with an engraving of a horse, bull or some sort of western motif. A new line dance started to form. Lynn and Jack tried their luck, "Come on, girls, let's go for a Madison dance."

"Oh please, it's out of the question right now. I never danced this in my whole life. Give me a chance to watch before I take the plunge," I replied in a panic.

"Okay, you two can sit this one out but we'll get you up for the next one," Lynn said laughing.

They put down their beers, strode out onto the dance floor and took their place in the front row where we could have clear view of their steps. The music started and we quickly saw that Jack and Lynn were brilliant dancers. They glided gracefully on the stage and I was surprised at the elegance of the choreography. The joyful energy was contagious and I felt the urge to join in.

Interestingly enough, western country dances were to become very popular in France in the years to come, so popular in fact that dance societies were formed that instituted rules, as in sports such as football or rugby, which imposed training courses for line dancing teachers and a state-approved diploma for anyone who wanted to give lessons or run clubs. I like to think Victorine and I were French western country dancing pioneers.

As soon as the dance finished, Lynn and Jack led us over to an empty area on the edge of the dance floor and began teaching us the steps.

"Step left foot forward, place right beside left and clap, step back on right foot, move left foot back and across the right, move left foot to the left, move left foot back and across the right . . . let's start again . . . Step left foot forward, place right beside left and clap, step back on right foot, move left foot back and across the right, move left foot to the left, move left foot back and across the right . . ."

I was doing my best but it wasn't coming easy. To make matters worse, Victorine, who had picked up the steps quickly, was dancing nimbly next to Jack and laughing loudly as she watched me.

"Maybe the problem is you're not wearing cowboy boots," she said as she executed an elegant turn.

I decided to ignore her and concentrate on my confused feet. I slowly made progress and my teacher rewarded my efforts by handing me another beer. I looked up and noticed that our odd quartet had drawn the attention of some curious onlookers, mostly girls gazing dreamily at our handsome partners. I was now feeling the effect of my two beers and I needed to run to the bathroom. Victorine joined me as we squeezed our way through the crowd, trying to find the restroom. I asked a passing waitress.

"Sure thang sugar, the ladies room is right there," she said, pointing to a sign that read "Heifers."

In the corner were two doors. One marked "Bulls", the other "Heifers."

"Okay, I guess "heifers" is the feminine for "bulls," said Victorine. *"Imagine that, toilets for women being called toilets for cows."*

"Well, I guess, Texan women don't mind being called cows," I said.

"I don't mind either. They're beautiful animals," replied Victorine. *"By the way, I guess you are liking Texas after all,"* she whispered.

I just shrugged and squeezed my way through the crowd.

The scene inside the surprisingly large ladies room was hilarious. I had never seen such a coquettish bunch of "heifers." Women were frantically fighting for space at the giant mirror, painstakingly applying new layers of foundation, making up their faces, spraying their hair, and dabbing on perfume. Inside their huge handbags they had packed their toiletry kits as if they were traveling. We were standing in their midst, waiting for an available toilet, totally fascinated by the mayhem when I noticed one of them eyeing us in the mirror. Despite her exasperation with her oily nose, she paused, then turned to look at us. I already knew which question she was going to ask.

"Y'all ain't from around here, are ya?"

"No, we're from Paris," we replied together.

"From PA-RIS!? Ama-zing!" she screamed.

This caught the attention of three curious girls who decided to join us. They were blonde, blue-eyed, big-breasted friendly girls, with cowboy boots. They started asking us questions all at once. Two beers had put me in a good mood and I was feeling a little silly in fact so I decided to get ahead of them.

"You want to know what it's like in Paris? Well, it's not Texas. You can search high and low in the stores along the Champs-Elysées but you can't find a decent pair of cowboy boots or cowboy hat. Worst of all, we have no cowboys, so we came here to get us some."

They burst into laughter but then "Chattahoochee" by Alan Jackson began booming from the dance floor and they shrieked happily.

"See you out there!" they shouted in unison and suddenly disappeared, reminding me of a swarm of butterflies.

Beneath their layers of make-up we found Texan women were incredibly friendly, endlessly smiling, even to other women, a refreshing change from the frosty demeanor of the French.

"*So, did you find out a little bit about Lynn?*" Victorine asked me.

"*I don't know anything about him but I'm starting to like the line dance!*" I answered rushing back to the dance floor.

I returned to find Lynn surrounded by giggling girls, batting their heavily mascaraed eyelashes. I looked down at my plain dress and sandals. Earlier I thought they looked simple and elegant. Now they seemed totally out of place. When Lynn looked up and saw me approaching, he smiled, stepped forward, and reached for my hand.

"Okay, are you ready to try a dance?" he asked, leading me to the dance floor.

Victorine didn't bother to wait for her dance partner. She jumped onto the dance floor and took her place in line; anxious to try out the new steps she had learned.

"One, two, three, four, five, six, seven, eight, right together, right together, step, turn, together, clap, left, together, left together, step, turn, together, clap, one two, three, four, five, six, seven, eight, cha-cha, front, cha-cha and back, one, two, three, four, five, six, seven, eight . . ."

It wasn't going smoothly and I was flip flapping in a panic. All those steps were too complicated for me and I was lost.

"I'm sorry. This one is a little too hard for me," I yelled over the music. "Can we go sit down?"

Lynn followed me to the bar where we found two empty stools. He took a long look at me as I caught my breath. I admired his finely chiseled nose and his dark blue eyes. He was handsome, Hollywood handsome, and his gentlemanly manners just added to his charm. If I meet his parents, I must compliment them, I thought.

"You are very different, you know . . . I kind of like it," he said looking out toward the dance floor and tapping his boot to the beat of the music.

I nodded. We were on the right track. Out on the dance floor, Victorine was making all the right steps and laughing up a storm with Jack. They waved at us to come back and join them. I declined with a wave of my hand. I was hoping Lynn was in the mood for confidences. I was intrigued by his dark good looks.

"You mean physically different?" I asked.

"Well, that too . . . and to tell you the truth, I'm kind of intimidated . . . I've never dated a French girl before." He took a sip of beer and continued looking toward the dance floor.

I laughed, a little nervously I must admit, touched by his sincerity but also wondering . . . were we on a date?

"Well, maybe I'm intimidated too. After all, you're like one of those mythic cowboys we see back at home in the films and I'm a French girl who has just made a fool of herself," I said.

At this he smiled, turned and looked at me intently. I nervously took a sip of my beer and looked out at Victorine laughing and twirling on the dance floor. As she had reminded me earlier, I knew nothing about this Texan and I yearned to open the door of his mind. I could feel Lynn's eyes on me.

"Say, this music is kinda loud. Would you like to walk outside where it's easier to talk?" asked Lynn. "It's a beautiful night."

"Yes," I said without hesitation.

As soon as we were outside, Lynn took my hand and said something about the beauty of the stars. My heart began beating faster and I quickly searched for something to say to quiet my nervousness.

"So, are you a real cowboy?" I asked, looking straight ahead as we slowly walked hand in hand across the parking lot.

"Well, actually, yes," he said with a little laugh. "My family owns a small cattle ranch where I mainly breed horses. I can take you and Victorine there tomorrow."

Instantly, my mind conjured up images of archetypal cowboys on horseback, riding the open range, sleeping under the stars, herding cattle and branding young calves with a hot iron. I wondered if these activities resembled those of a modern day cowboy. I pictured Victorine prancing inside on the dance floor with Jack and imagined her excitement when she heard of our invitation. It could wait. I was enjoying myself and wanted to savor the moment.

"Well, yes," I said. "I . . . I mean . . . we would like that . . . very much."

I felt a soft tug on my hand and realized Lynn had stopped walking and we were now standing next to his pickup truck. He turned to face me and gently put both his arms around my waist. I barely knew this cowboy and yet, he was going to kiss me—there was no question about it now. Yes, I was physically attracted to him, we had had a couple of dances but we hadn't yet bonded in a conversation. In fact, we had almost no conversation to speak of. I didn't know anything about his tastes, hobbies, family or his childhood but I was as excited as a schoolgirl. When I lifted my face to look up into his magnificent blue eyes I decided none of this really mattered so much after all. My eyes closed and I felt his strong soft lips press against mine as his arms tightened around me.

"NATASHA! There you are. We have been looking for you EVERYWHERE!"

My eyes flew open and I unlocked my lips from Lynn's. Victorine was standing before us, hands on hips, looking at me reprovingly. Jack was behind her, snickering. He winked at Lynn.

"You disappeared. How smart is that? I was about to call the police. I thought something happened to you."

"Well, as you can see, I'm alive," I said, then switching to English for the benefit of Lynn and Jack, "We were just taking a walk, admiring the beautiful stars."

Victorine takes her role as big sister very seriously but she could be such a harpy when she's stressed. I was fuming. Every fiber of my being longed to get back to that moment of intimacy but it was now ruined. Lynn was sweetly apologizing to Victorine but I was in no mood to follow his lead. I looked at Jack and said, "Did you notice the stars are particularly beautiful tonight, Jack? Did you know that Victorine just loves to look at the stars? If you ask her nicely maybe she can even point out the Crab Nebula!"

"Forget the stars. Let's go!" Victorine barked like a drill sergeant.

The tension in the cab of the pickup was palpable as we drove back to our rental car. Neither Victorine nor I said a word as we both stared straight ahead. Finally, Lynn broke the silence.

"Say, Victorine," he said, "I invited Natasha out to our family's ranch tomorrow. I was hoping you'd like to come along?"

She tried to ignore him but her curiosity got the better of her.

"Ranch? Oh really? Well, what sort of ranch?" she asked, trying to act blasé.

"Well, it's a cattle ranch mainly but I'm in charge of breeding and training our horses. You have to have a good horse under you when it comes time to round up the cattle. I have a few prize Quarter horses I'd love you to meet," he said, taking his eyes from the road and turning to smile at both of us. That was it, the magic words. The moment Victorine learned she was going to the ranch of an authentic cowboy my sin was forgiven. As for myself, I couldn't stay mad at my sister for long. As annoying as it was, her overprotective nature came from her sincere concern for my safety. By the time we reached the Armadillo Diner we were all laughing and had finalized our plans for tomorrow's visit to Lynn's family ranch. As we watched our two cowboys drive out of the parking lot she said to me, *"I totally understand you wanting to slip off to kiss him, but next time, make sure you tell me where to find you, OK?"*

Mona's Shrimp and Cheesy Grits
Serves 4

- 1 cup coarsely ground grits
- 3 cups water
- 1 cup whole milk
- 1cup grated Parmesan cheese
- 1 tablespoon fresh lemon juice
- 1 tablespoon salt
- 1 teaspoon freshly ground black pepper
- 1 onion, chopped
- 1 leek, minced
- 1 tablespoon finely minced garlic
- 3 tablespoons butter
- 2 tablespoon olive oil
- 1 pound shrimp, peeled and deveined
- 1 tablespoon fresh chopped parsley

1. Bring 3 cups of water to a boil in a large saucepan over medium-high heat.
2. Stir in the salt and reduce the heat to medium low. Cook, stirring frequently 25 to 30 minutes until they are thick and the grains are tender.
3. Stir in the milk and cook and stir 5 minutes more.
4. While the grits are cooking, heat 1 tablespoon of the butter and olive oil in a large skillet over medium high heat until hot.
5. Add the onion, leek with the shrimps and stir until the shrimp are cooked. Add the garlic and lemon juice and cook and stir one minute more. Remove from the heat and set aside.
6. When the grits are tender add the remaining butter and the Parmesan cheese and season with salt and pepper; stir to mix and melt cheese. Add a little more milk if they are not creamy enough.
7. Place on individual plates and top with shrimp. Sprinkle the parsley on top. Serve warm topped with additional Parmesan cheese if desired.

Vegetarian Cactus Chili
Serves 6 to 8

- ½ lb fresh nopalitos, nopales prickly pear cactus paddles that have been stripped of spines, cleaned, and chopped
- 5 ripe tomatoes, chopped, or use one 1 can diced tomatoes (15oz)
- 1 can (24 oz) tomato sauce
- 1 can of black beans (15 oz)
- 1 can of corn (15 oz)
- 2 fresh onions, chopped
- 6 garlic cloves, minced
- 1 Jalapeno pepper, stem and seeds removed, chopped
- 3 tablespoons of olive oil
- 3 tablespoons of fresh cilantro
- ½ cup chili powder
- ¼ cup of cumin powder
- Sea salt and freshly ground pepper

1. Heat olive oil in a large sauté pan on medium high heat.
2. Add onions, garlic, and jalapeño.
3. Sauté for a few minutes, stirring occasionally.
4. Add nopalitos and sauté for several more minutes.
5. Add chopped tomatoes and tomato sauce.
6. Stir well and lower the heat.
7. Add black beans, corn, chili and cumin powder.
8. Add sea salt and freshly ground pepper to taste.
9. Bring to simmer and cook for 30 minutes over low heat stirring often.
10. Serve with cilantro, cheddar and sour cream for topping over rice.

Steak Tartare
Serves 4

- 1 pound beef tenderloin (finely ground, preferably grass fed)
- 2 tablespoons Dijon mustard
- ½ cup capers
- 4 cornichons (gherkins finely chopped)
- 1 cup of minced shallots
- 1 tablespoon Tabasco sauce
- 1 tablespoon of Worcestershire sauce
- 4 tablespoons of Cognac
- 1 bunch of fresh parsley, chopped
- 4 egg yolks
- 1 tablespoon of olive oil
- salt and fresh ground pepper

1. In a bowl, mix the meat with some of the parsley, the Worcestershire sauce, the Cognac, the Tabasco sauce, the Dijon mustard, and salt and pepper.
2. Form the mixture into 4 round patties.
3. The remaining ingredients should be arranged around the meat, and an egg yolk placed in the center of each serving. This allows everyone to add and mix and season to their taste.
4. You can also serve the patties cooked. Heat the olive oil in a large non-stick frying pan and cook the patties for 3–4 minutes on each side to your liking.

Chapter Four

Sacred Cows

The next morning we awoke to another glorious day, unaware of the huge disappointment awaiting us. After breakfast we located a pay phone and I called Larry Fitzgerald, the spokesman in charge of the media for the Texas Department of Criminal Justice.

"Hello? Mr. Fitzgerald? Good morning, this is Natasha Saulnier. I'm calling to confirm our appointment on Monday," I said, in my best businesslike tone of voice reserved for bureaucrats. "I believe we have an appointment scheduled for two p.m."

"Yes, good morning Ms. Saulnier," he said. "Let me see, let me see."

I could hear the papers rustling on his desk behind his heavy breathing.

"Ah yes, I have your paperwork right here. I have you down for a two p.m. interview. I can give you forty minutes of my time." he said.

"Good," I answered, "and will you be escorting us to the Terrel death row unit after the interview?"

There was pause and I felt a chill coming from his end of the line.

"Ah, no Ms. Saulnier," he said, "I've gone over your paperwork and you won't be granted access to Terrel unit. We've found the European media presents the least objective reporting, showing little to no regard for victims' rights, and frankly," a venomous tone now in his voice, "I dislike French journalists most of all."

Astonishment and anger involuntarily exploded from my lips.

"What are you talking about? . . . but . . . in your letter you wrote that we would be . . ."

"Thank you Ms. Saulnier," he said, cutting me off. "I will see you Monday at 2 p.m."

There was a loud click in my earpiece and I stood there in shock, listening to the buzz of the dial tone, my mouth open in disbelief. I repeatedly pounded the handset down onto the cradle. It bounced off and hung there, swinging in the warm breeze.

"What, what did he say, what did he say?" Victorine kept repeating but I was too upset to answer.

I was mortified. I didn't care at all about Larry Fitzgerald's scripted answers. Yes, it was going to be interesting to talk to Farley Matchett and LaRoyce Smith, I already knew that the interview would be strictly supervised, but the visit to the death row unit was supposed to be the highlight of the reportage. This was terrible. What was I going to tell my editor? As my anger and shock slowly subsided, I recounted the conversation to Victorine. We decided to wait before breaking the bad news to our editor. After all, there was still a chance a miracle might happen. Besides, we were looking forward to our visit to Lynn's ranch and didn't want to let our bad news ruin the rest of the day.

Lynn and Jack arrived at our campground at ten a.m. When they peeked inside our tent they looked at each other, shook their heads and laughed.

"What's so funny?" asked Victorine.

"You brought this tent and your sleeping bags on the airplane?" asked Jack.

"Yes, what's so strange about that?" I asked.

Jack shook his head.

"Well dang. When I think of French girls I think of perfume and, and . . . well I don't know what I think of but, I don't think of tents and sleeping bags and campfires for sure," he said. "My Mama thought you were staying at the Hilton."

"Your Mama?" Victorine asked, arching her eyebrow.

I turned to look at Lynn.

"And where did your parents think we were staying?" I asked.

"Come on, we better get movin'," he said, opening the door of the pickup.

As we drove down the highway, leaving mini-malls and filling stations behind us, the landscape became greener and we were soon passing beautiful pastures filled with grazing cattle.

"Our spread starts about here. There's some of our herd up over there," said Lynn, pointing toward a field to the right with scattered clusters of cows. As we passed, a few of them stopped grazing and lifted their heads to watch us.

"Are we almost there?" asked Victorine, leaning forward to get a better view through the windshield.

"No, not quite," said Jack. He looked over at Lynn and grinned.

"They're beautiful," said Victorine.

Lynn slowed the truck and we turned right onto a gravel road that passed through a beautiful white wrought iron entrance gate with the words "Elmwood Hill Ranch" arching over the top. The truck's tires kicked up dust behind us as we bounced down a winding gravel road shaded by giant oak and elm trees. Huge pastures stretched out beyond on either side. After a few minutes Victorine asked Lynn if he had lost his way. I laughed but the two cowboys just smiled. We had been driving for a while and now I was curious.

"How big is your ranch?" I asked, spotting a house in the distance beyond the trees.

"It's about twenty thousand acres," said Lynn as he waved to two riders on horseback coming the opposite direction. Victorine turned to watch them as we passed.

I was trying to do the math in my head. Let's see, if one acre is approximately point four hectares, that would be . . .

"That's about eight thousand hectares," said Victorine, "That's enormous."

"No, no," said Lynn, "Here in Texas ranches aren't considered big till you get up over one hundred thousand acres. But I will say, we make good use of the land we've got."

Victorine looked at me. The expression on her face said it all. She was impressed.

We rounded a curve and in front of us stood a massive two story white antebellum mansion. Four columns supported a triangular portico over the entrance and two large wings extended from either side. I counted over a dozen windows and two brick chimneys rising at either end. Gorgeous pink magnolia trees and huge oaks surrounded the mansion. Victorine kept silent. Although not nearly as grand as the numerous country estates we knew in France, it was an impressive private residence.

We stepped out of the truck and Lynn led us along a gravel path to the rear of the house. I noticed an older couple, I guessed to be Lynn's parents, waiting for us on a large flower-covered terrace next to a swimming pool. I started to feel slightly uncomfortable. We were obviously expected. I wondered what exactly they were expecting. The white-haired man, I judged to be in his sixties, wearing a striped light gray flannel suit with an American eagle bolo tie, a big silver buckle belt, and a white cowboy hat, studied us carefully as we approached. The short-haired blonde woman, I guessed to be slightly younger, wearing a flower print summer dress and floppy sun hat, turned to welcome us with a pleasant smile.

"Mama, Papa, I'd like to introduce you to Natasha and Victorine, the two reporters from France I told you about. They're here to write a story on Texas prisons," Lynn said, turning to me with a reassuring smile.

"Well hello Natasha, hello Victorine," the woman said, stepping forward and gently shaking our hands. "It's a pleasure to meet you. I've heard such nice things about you from Lynn. My name is Vernetta and this is my husband Richard."

The man stepped forward, grabbed my hand and pumped it hard.

"No need to be so formal. You just call me Dick," he said with a big grin. He continued to hold my hand but took a half step back and looked me up and down.

"So you're the little French filly my son's taken a shine to," he said.

I felt my face flush as he looked at Lynn and winked. He finally released my hand and turned to Victorine.

"Vicktoreen, pleasure to meet you, call me Dick," he said, grabbing her hand and pumping it too.

"So, you're here to write a story about our correctional system?" he asked. "Well that's fine, mighty fine. We're sure proud of it. Finest in the nation, hell, the world I reckon. I guess you two are here to take a few notes so you can teach them a thing or two back home."

I looked at Victorine and could see she was beginning to bristle.

"Well actually, we're here to . . ." Victorine started to speak but I jumped in nervously to interrupt her before she could ruffle any feathers.

"What a wonderful property you have. It reminds me of J.R. Ewing's Southfork ranch. All of France fell in love with Texas after watching 'Dallas,'" I said in a panic.

Dick let out a huge belly laugh. Victorine glared at me.

"Well, I'm no J.R. Ewing," said Dick, "but we're doing okay here."

"Well, it's a pleasure to meet you but y'all better get started," said Vernetta, "I'm sure Dick and the boys have a lot to show you. I'll have Maria prepare some tea and a snack for you when you're finished."

Dick put his arm around my shoulder and walked me past a large barn alongside an enormous pasture. His tone turned serious.

"Our family has been in the cattle business for five generations, since way back before Texas was even a state. I hope you like cows 'cause I'm going to show you some of the finest Angus cows in the country," said Dick. He was a proud Texan.

Lynn and Jack followed while Victorine lagged behind, silently taking photos. I braced myself for her inevitable comments. Victorine had become a vegetarian years earlier while living in London, studying for her degree in Environmental Sciences. One of her university lectures detailed the beef industry's production practices leading up to Great Britain's first outbreak of "Mad Cow" disease in 1986. In the middle of it something inside her clicked and in that moment she became vegetarian.

"Natsha, you have to stop eating meat," she lectured me the next time I came to visit her in London. *"The beef in the markets now is not like it*

use to be. Not like Maman bought when we were small. You have no idea what's in it now . . . growth hormones, antibiotics, and, listen to this, they grind up cow bones and offal . . . then add it to their feed . . . their making them cannibals Natasha, cannibals! It's crazy! Cows are supposed to eat grass, not each other."

What she said was absolutely true and her fears were not unfounded. Indeed, when the outbreak went public, British beef was immediately banned throughout Europe and although the restrictions were lifted a short time later in other countries, France continued the boycott for twelve years. Reports and debates on the safety and purity of beef were constantly in the French media and everyone in the country had their own opinion. Fortunately, our mother bought her beef from a trusted local farmer she had known for decades and never let the fear of Mad Cow disease enter her kitchen. One afternoon for lunch, during the following Christmas holiday when Victorine was home from university, our mother prepared one of her specialties, steak tartare: finely ground beef tenderloin mixed with parsley, Worcestershire sauce, Tabasco sauce, Dijon mustard, salt, pepper, and Cognac. The mélange of ingredients is then formed into patties and served raw with a raw egg yolk on top.

"Yuck," cried Victorine when she entered the kitchen and saw what our mother was making, "I'm not eating that."

"VIC-TOR-INE," our mother snapped, "I don't want to hear it."

Ever since her arrival Victorine had been rabidly lecturing the entire family about her newfound vegetarianism. After a week of the constant tirade our mother's patience was growing thin. Papa, our mother's loyal sous-chef, was sitting at the table with me peeling carrots. Still a bit bemused by Victorine's culinary about-face, he tried to reason with her.

"Victorine, this beef is from the Kervalguen farm outside Brest. You can't find better anywhere," he said, "I picked it up yesterday, and look what else grandfather Kervalguen gave me."

His eyes twinkled as he wiped his hands on his dish-towel, reached into the cabinet over his head and pulled out a bottle filled with a beautiful amber liquid: a bottle of homemade hard cider from the Kervalguen farm. He pinched his fingers to his lips, gave them a loud kiss, then spread them wide to toss it into the air. Grandfather Kervalguen and our grand-father had been good friends and our father had known him since he was a small boy. The community of local farmers and horsemen like our father was small and it was nearly impossible for them to pay a visit, even on business, without sitting down to share stories and a drink.

"*They aren't one of those 'factory farms' you keep talking about,*" he said, "*They been on that land for who knows how many generations and . . .*"

"*I don't care,*" Victorine said interrupting him, "*We shouldn't be eating meat. I now believe like the Hindus that the cow is sacred.*"

Our mother let out an uncontrolled laugh.

"*Oh, so now you're a Hindu?*" she asked.

"*No, but it makes sense to revere the cow,*" she answered. "*You keep a cow and she gives her milk freely. With it you make yogurt and cheese and a family can eat for her entire lifetime, but, you kill the cow to eat her flesh and she feeds you for maybe a few weeks, then she's gone and you starve.*"

"*So, when was the last time you milked a cow?*" asked our mother.

"*That's not the point,*" Victorine shot back, "*You don't understand . . .*"

As they continued arguing I watched Papa slowly rise from his chair and place the bowl of peeled carrots on the counter. Then I watched him quietly open the door of the spice cabinet behind Victorine. He peered inside, pulled out a jar of red curry, opened it, dipped his finger inside then quickly reached from behind and dabbed a big red dot in the middle of Victorine's forehead.

"*Okay, Shiva,*" he said, "*you eat your salad and we'll finish your steak.*"

We all laughed except for Victorine who looked at us through nar-rowed eyes, shook her head, and stormed out of the kitchen mumbling to herself. The three of us sat down to eat Maman's delicious steak tartare while Victorine sulked in her room.

My thoughts were suddenly jerked back to the moment by the sound of Dick's voice shouting orders in Spanish to a group of workers in the field. They acknowledged with a wave, mounted their waiting horses and rode off. I looked around and saw hundreds of hornless sturdy black cows grazing in the surrounding pastures.

"You see, girls, our cows are lucky. They live in what I like to call our bovine country club," said Dick, chuckling at his own wit and waiting for my acknowledgement.

"Oh really, I don't recall being hung upside down and having my throat slit last time I went to a spa, do you Natasha?" Victorine said snapping a photo. She moved her eye from the lens to Dick, forced a laugh and an insincere smile. Thank goodness he didn't understand French. With a puzzled look on his face he smiled and continued.

"We grow only certified Angus beef here. Notice they don't have any horns? They're very different from your Normandes. This breed originally came from Scotland and was brought to Kansas in the eighteen hundreds. At first they were called 'freaks' and the ranchers wanted nothin' to do with them but when they noticed how hardy they were and how quickly they grew, they warmed up to them right quick."

"Do they only eat grass?" I asked.

I looked over at Lynn who was smiling at me, making it difficult to concentrate on what Dick was saying.

"Mostly, but we also feed them corn and other grains mixed with supplements and low level antibiotics to make sure they leave the ranch as soon as possible."

I looked at Victorine who was wincing. I held my breath, hoping she wouldn't poison the congenial atmosphere with one of her vegetarian tirades. Now I saw our mythic cowboy was the son of a high profit beef producer. Not so romantic after all.

"How long do they stay on your ranch?" I asked.

"They leave here anywhere from between six and twelve months old. Then they go to the feed-lot. When a calf is born, it weighs sixty to one hundred pounds. They are weaned at six to ten months when they weigh in the range of four hundred fifty to seven hundred pounds. Once they reach market weight, which is between twelve hundred to fourteen hundred pounds at about eighteen to twenty-two months of age, they are sent to a processing facility to be harvested."

"Harvested?" Victorine asked, pouring all her disgust into her one word question.

"Yes, slaughtered," answered Dick.

I looked at Lynn. He seemed confident in his own environment and was looking at me with an intensity that made me a little uncomfortable.

"*How sad,*" Victorine said, looking away from the cows. I knew my sister and I suspected a lecture was brewing inside her, thinking of the best way to "educate" her hosts. I braced myself for the inevitable confrontation. What came next from her lips I wasn't expecting.

"*Well,*" she said bitterly, "*Maybe they'll get lucky, get ground up into a Nathan's hot dog and help Joey Chesnut win next year's trophy.*"

Dick looked at both of us with a puzzled expression. By this time Victorine had stopped trying to hide her disgust. Dick recognized it, nodded and said, "Ah, I understand. You two delicate flowers don't like to talk about slaughtering animals. Lynn, why don't you show them your domain? I wanna see a happy smile on these beautiful girls' faces. Excuse me ladies but right now I've got to go talk over some business with Hector our foreman, but I wanna hear all about your reporting on our prisons when I get back."

Dick walked over to a pickup truck parked near the barn, climbed in and sped off down a gravel road, disappearing in a cloud of dust. His last words unnerved me. That positive spin on our story I was searching for was still eluding me. Maybe I could say we had come all the way from France to report on the Texas prison infrastructure? I remembered reading a report on the unhealthy conditions in French prisons.

"Your father is very nice," I said to Lynn, "a real gentleman."

Jack let out a sudden involuntary laugh.

"Well, I've never heard him called that," said Lynn, turning to look at Jack, "but they sure broke the mold when they made him."

"*Really? I hope so,*" said Victorine, who then flashed a sweet smile.

Lynn took my hand and led me to another fenced pasture where several horses were peacefully grazing. Victorine and Jack followed. The four of us rested our elbows on the fence rail, silently watching the horses in the field. I looked over at Victorine and saw some of the tension leave her body. She was at home and happy when she was around horses. A hawk circled overhead framed by a passing cloud.

"You see the beautiful palomino Quarter horse over there? His name is Tank. He's not a youngster but he can still work cattle," said Lynn.

"He's beautiful," said Victorine "but I have my eye on that Appaloosa."

"Yes, her name is Penny. She was born right here on the ranch," said Lynn.

"She looks like she has some Arab blood," said Victorine.

"Yes, we call this breed the Araloosa," said Lynn turning to Victorine with a look of surprise, "It's a cross between a Arabian and an Apaloosa. You have an eye for horses, Victorine."

"She grew up on horses," I said, "Our father is a horse trader like our grandfather and Victorine spent her childhood with him working for the family's equestrian club."

"Penny reminds me of Sitou, my Appaloosa," said Victorine.

"She had a foal last year. There she is, that leopard spotted beauty," said Lynn.

"Wow, impressive head," said Victorine, "she has the elegance of an aristocrat."

"Yes, she reminds me of a French girl," said Lynn.

He turned to me and lowered his voice. "Her name is Moonlight Kiss."

I looked into his gorgeous blue eyes and my heart began to pound. He took my hand, gave it a soft squeeze, then looked out to the pasture and made a clicking sound with his tongue. The foal looked up and trotted over to Lynn. He reached into his pocket, pulled out a piece of carrot, and offered it to her. She took it from him, let him pat her nose softly, then walked back to the field.

"She's my favorite," he whispered softly in my ear. I felt my cheeks flush and suddenly forgot about Dick and the lies I planned to tell him.

We returned to the terrace were we found Vernetta seated at the head of a long glass-topped wrought iron table, shaded beneath a wisteria covered arbor. As we approached, she picked up and rang a small bell then placed it back on the table.

"I thought y'all might be thirsty after paradin' around in that hot sun," said Vernetta. "I asked Maria to fix some tea."

"Thank you, Mama," said Lynn.

He leaned over to give his mother a kiss on the check then pulled out the chair directly to her left and motioned me to sit.

"Yes, thank you," I echoed as I sat down.

Jack, who had begun seating himself to Vernetta's right, sprang up just as his rear end was about to hit the cushion and offered it to Victorine. Victorine pulled out the chair next to him and sat down.

A plump middle-aged Mexican woman appeared carrying a tray with a large pitcher and glasses filled with ice. She placed it on the table in front of Vernetta then disappeared.

"So, did y'all have a nice tour of our ranch?" Vernetta asked pouring a glass of iced tea and handing it to me.

"Natasha and Victorine grew up on a horse farm, Mama," said Lynn.

"Oh, really, that's nice," said Vernetta, obviously unimpressed. She continued filling glasses of tea and passing them around the table.

Maria returned to the table with another large tray. On it were two wooden bowls filled with triangular bite-sized chips and a number of smaller ceramic bowls, some filled with a red sauce and others filled with a sauce the unmistakable color of avocado.

"Mmm, what's that," asked Victorine.

"This is Maria's salsa and guacamole," said Lynn placing one bowl of chips between me and him and the other between Victorine and Jack. He dipped a corner of one of the chips into the red salsa and popped it in his mouth.

"Here, try some," he said placing two bowls in front of me.

I dipped a chip into the bowl of red salsa and took a bite. Suddenly all my taste buds were shouting . . . Spicy . . . Tangy . . . Delicious.

"Mmm, the salsa is delicious," I said, "and so are the chips. They taste so fresh."

"Yup, Maria makes her own corn chips from scratch," said Jack crunching one in his mouth.

"Now try the guacamole," said Lynn pushing the other bowl closer.

I scooped up a dab of the green avocado dip and took a bite. I was no stranger to avocados. At home we would slice them in half, remove the stone, sprinkle on some salt and eat them with a spoon like a melon, but this, this was heavenly. I could taste tomato, onion, garlic and was that lime that gave it its bite? I looked across the table. Victorine had pulled the bowl of chips in front of her along with a bowl of each of the dips and was alternating scooping and munching from each like a machine. Lynn and Jack looked at each other and began to laugh.

"You never had Tex-Mex food before?" asked Jack, a note of surprise in his voice.

Victorine looked up with eyes wide, shook her head as she continued eating.

"No," I answered. "It's wonderful. My mouth feels like it's on fire but I can't wait for the next bite."

Victorine finished scraping the last bit of guacamole from her bowl and sat back in her chair with a contented sigh.

"Wow, I've heard of Tex-Mex food but never tried it," she said.

Vernetta sat sipping her tea looking serene and content.

"Lynn," she said, "Why don't you and Jack take the girls to El Coyote for dinner. Order them some quesadillas, enchiladas, fajitas . . . give them the full Tex-Mex tour."

Victorine's eyes grew wide and she nodded yes.

Maria's Guacamole Dip

Serves 6 to 8

- 4 ripe avocados
- 1 small tomato, coarsely chopped
- ¼ cup peeled, finely chopped white onion
- 1 jalapeño seeded and minced
- 1 garlic clove finely diced
- 4 tablespoons finely chopped fresh cilantro
- juice of ½ fresh lime
- 1 teaspoon of paprika
- Salt and fresh ground pepper

1. Cut the avocados in half, twist to remove the pit, scoop out the pulp, place in a medium-size bowl and mash the avocado with a fork so that the mixture is a bit chunky.
2. Combine half the onions, half the garlic, half the jalapeño, and half the cilantro in a mortar or food processor, season with about ½ tsp. salt, then grind or pulse into a smooth paste.
3. Transfer the paste and the avocado into a serving bowl. Mix well with a wooden spoon and stir in remaining onions, jalapeño, and cilantro, then gently mix in the chopped tomatoes.
4. Sprinkle the fresh lime juice and the paprika over the dip and mix well.
5. Taste and add salt. Add pepper and more seasonings if necessary.

Beignets de Carnaval
Serves 4 to 6

- 3 cups of all-purpose flour
- ½ cup of sugar
- 4 eggs (preferably organic or free-range)
- 1 pinch of salt
- 1 teaspoon baking powder
- ½ butter, softened
- ¼ cup confectioners' sugar

1. Pour the flour and salt into a bowl and make a crater. Into the crater put the eggs, sugar, and the butter.
2. Mix well with a wooden spoon, then turn out of bowl onto a heavily floured surface.
3. Knead until mixture is a firm dough. Let stand, covered, for 1 hour.
4. Roll out dough till it reaches a thickness of ¼ inch. Cut the dough in different shapes.
5. Fry in 360°F hot oil until the beignets pop up and become brown.
6. Drain onto paper towels.
7. Shake confectioners' sugar on hot beignets. Serve warm.

Chapter Five

Rodeo Daze

S unset approached, day glided smoothly into evening and we were
able to escape from Elmwood Hill Ranch without incident. Luckily,
Dick was called away to attend to some business on a far corner of
the sprawling ranch and we finished our visit sipping unbearably sweet
iced tea on the terrace with Vernetta who was content keeping the conversation confined to nothing more than pleasantries.

Jack and Lynn brought us to a trendy spot for drinks where they introduced us to their friends. Everywhere we went, as soon as we disclosed
our origins, we triggered the same reaction we got from the "heifers" in
the restroom at the dancehall. "From PA-RIS, FRANCE? A-MA-ZING!"
Victorine and I exchanged glances confirming we had come to the same
conclusion; these two cowboys were taking us out to show us off. Maybe
we were really just a couple of prize "heifers" ourselves. The Texan
men we spoke with seemed to have the attitude, "Once you've been to
Texas, why go anywhere else," but the Texan women, excited to have two
Parisiennes in their midst, were eager to discuss fashion and the latest
French designers. They were soon disappointed. Haute couture is the last
thing Victorine and I think about, so when we steered the conversation

about fashion towards what was truly of interest to us, the deplorable conditions of the child labor force in the garment industry's Asian sweat-shops, their eyes began to glaze over and they excused themselves to go back to chatting and laughing with their friends. Like Jack, I imagine their image of French women was different than what they had in front of them.

Jack and Lynn followed Vernetta's suggestion and brought us to El Coyote, an upscale Tex-Mex restaurant with a menu filled with vegetarian choices for Victorine. She repaid their thoughtfulness by refraining from making any comments about the huge steaks the waitress placed in front of them.

"Jack, does your family have a ranch too?" asked Victorine.

"No, his daddy's a big oil man, Jack's gonna be one too, provided he can swim," said Lynn looking at Jack with a grin.

"Oil? I thought you were both cowboys," said Victorine.

Lynn let out a big laugh.

"Hell, he can barely ride a horse," said Lynn

"Swim? What do you mean swim? Swim in oil?" I asked.

"No, not in oil," said Jack. "My grand-daddy was a wildcatter who was lucky and hit it big back in. . ."

"Wild cat?" I asked, "what kind of wild cat?"

"Shush," said Victorine. "Stop interrupting and listen."

"No, that's alright," said Jack, "I'll explain. A wildcatter is what they call someone who leases a piece of land, then sets up a drilling rig on it to search for oil. Back in my grand-daddy's day, Texas was filled with men just like him who would beg, borrow or steal enough money to finance a rig in the hopes of drillin' down and hittin' oil. Nine times out of ten they would hit nothin' or maybe just water. That's what happened to my grand-daddy, twice, and then on his third try he hit oil. Lucky thing too because by then he was up to his neck in debt."

"What a story," said Victorine. "He was lucky."

"Shoot," said Lynn, "lucky's not even the word for it. Go on Jack, tell them the whole story."

"They don't want to hear an old story like that," said Jack shaking his head.

"Yes we do," said Victorine as we both nodded eagerly. "Well, okay," he said. "Like I was sayin', he was out of money and so in debt to everybody that no one would even give him the time of day. He had set up a rig on a piece of land he leased outside of Midland, west of here. He was down over four thousand feet when he ran out of drill pipe. Without it he couldn't go any deeper. Stuck between a rock and a hard place, he was desperate. Well, he knew that over the nearby ridge there was another rig with a crew of three other wildcatters. He drove his truck over, parked it behind the ridge out of sight, crept up closer to get a better look and saw that two of the men had gone for supplies and a night out in town. After dark, he snuck into their camp, came up behind the man who stayed behind to guard the rig. He hit him on the back of the head with a lead pipe, knocked him out and tied him up. Then he drove his truck in, loaded up as much pipe as he could and drove back to his rig and went back to drilling all night."

"This is the best part," said Lynn, "listen."

"Well, like I said," continued Jack, "he drilled all night and come day-break, when the two returned to their rig, found their partner tied up and a load of pipe missing, it didn't take them long to figure out what happened. They followed the tire tracks over the ridge to my grand-daddy's place. When they saw him and their load of pipe they didn't bother askin' questions, they just drove in and started shootin'. My grand-daddy grabbed his rifle, took cover and started shootin' back. They were in a standoff and my grand-daddy was sure he was a goner when all of sudden there was a rumbling deep underground. The night's drilling had done the trick. One by one lengths of drill pipe came shooting out of the ground. The well blew-in, one of the biggest gushers anyone had seen for years. Oil started raining down on him. He ran out and started jumping and dancing, covered head to toe in black Texas crude."

Victorine and I looked at each other wide-eyed, amazed at the incredible story.

"Didn't they shoot him then? He stole their equipment!" I said.

"Hell no," said Jack, "they were all wildcatters, happy to see any well come in. Besides, it doesn't make sense to shoot a man who's just become a millionaire. They knew he'd pay 'em back. Sure, the guy with the bump on his head was a little sore but it he didn't stay mad for long. A year later he was best man at my grand-daddy's wedding and a year after was named my daddy's godfather."

"That story gets better every time I hear it," said Lynn, raising his glass. "To Texas wildcatters!"

"To Texas wildcatters," repeated Jack, joining him in the toast.

"But, I'm still confused," I said. "Why do you have to swim?"

Lynn and Jack looked at each other and laughed.

"Lynn's just jokin'," said Jack, "My grand-daddy brought my daddy into the business, but he made him learn it from the ground up. He had to work as a rough-neck on the rigs to start out and now I'm doing the same. I work on one of our company's oil platforms in the Gulf of Mexico."

"Are you on vacation?" asked Victorine.

"Sort of," said Jack. "The crew schedule working on oil platforms is three weeks on, three weeks off. I decided to come up to and see Lynn during this break."

"Yep, there's always a bunk at the ranch for Jack," said Lynn looking at Jack and nodding.

"So, a cowboy and an oil man, how do you two know each other?" I asked.

"University . . . Texas A&M. We were fraternity brothers and room-mates," said Lynn, "three out of our four years. Yup, we raised a little hell."

Lynn and Jack exchanged a glance between themselves and I found myself wondering what these two young Texans considered "a little hell."

After dinner, our two escorts took us back to the Midnight Rodeo. It was Saturday night and the dance floor was more crowded than the night before, which just added to the fun. I was relaxed and the line dance steps were coming to me more easily. Soon I was feeling a little "in-Texa-cated." When Lynn asked if I'd like to step outside for some fresh air, I nodded yes and whispered to Victorine that I'd be back soon and left her on the dance floor kicking and stomping with Jack. Outside, Lynn took my hand and we walked to his pickup where he pulled a blanket out of the cab, climbed up and lay it down on the floor of the back bed of the truck. He then bent down, put his hands around my waist, and I felt his muscles tighten under his shirt as he gently lifted me up into the back. We sat down, our legs stretched out, our backs resting against the inside of the truck bed. I looked up into his eyes and he kissed me gently but firmly. My body relaxed as a warm rush ran from my lips to my toes. Thankfully our second moonlight kiss transpired without any interruption. He put his arm around me and I lay my head on his shoulder as we looked up at the stars and I listened to the muffled sound of music from inside the club.

"I guess this is as good a time as any to ask," he said. "Do you have a boyfriend back home?"

"You mean back home in France?" I asked.

"Well, back home in France or New York," he said.

"No and no," I said, "I was so busy working and studying at university I didn't have time to even think about a relationship."

"Not even dating anyone?" He asked.

"I'm not sure what you mean by 'dating,'" I said.

"You know, dating . . . going out on a date," he said.

"That doesn't help me understand," I said.

"Okay, if I had to give you a fancy dictionary definition it would be, well, when two people date, uh, they're trying to ascertain whether or not they are compatible for a relationship and, uh, possibly marriage, yeah, that's it, that's dating," he answered.

I looked up at the stars.

"When two people date . . . Hmm, how about when three people date," I said turning to look at him with a playful smile.

"What?' he said, sitting up quickly and looking at me quizzically.

I laughed and put my hand on his cheek.

"I'm just teasing you, having fun," I said, "I guess I don't date then. When I go out with a man, I just try to enjoy my time with him without thinking of marriage. It has to be more natural than that. Otherwise, it takes away from the fun of discovering somebody spontaneously," I answered.

"So, there's no rules at all?" he asked, his eyes growing wide.

He seemed surprised so I answered honestly.

"No, my only rule is spontaneity and pleasure . . ." I answered.

By "pleasure," I meant "fun" but as I was saying it I realized that to an American ear, it might have connotations of sexual pleasure. I quickly added, " . . . which doesn't mean French women sleep with all the men they go out with or that French men are all hot rabbits."

I turned my head and looked up into his eyes.

"And how about you? Are you dating anyone?" I asked. "I saw a few pretty cowgirls inside who had their eyes on you while you were dancing."

"Right now, I'm with you," he answered.

His arms tightened around me and I melted into his embrace. We kissed deeply for a long moment then sat back and watched the stars as we listened to the music, my head on his shoulder, his fingers twirling a lock of my hair.

I hadn't been held in the arms of a man for a long time and had almost forgotten how comfortable it could feel. I had been so absorbed in my research, busy working on that damned exam, reading and writing about the lives of others that I'd forgotten to live myself. And what did I get for my efforts? Nothing. The rejection was such a disappointment that I had to get away, and where did I find myself now? In a place where people not only live, they live big. Yes, everything was bigger in Texas. Why had I fallen so hard for this cowboy? Was I making up for lost time? It didn't matter right now. This felt good. It felt right.

I felt Lynn's warmth next to me and the rise and fall of his chest. I buried myself deeper into his embrace, his breath on my cheek.

"Stay with me tonight," he whispered in my ear.

My body tightened and I sat up quickly.

I laughed nervously, thinking how to answer, what to say.

"I . . . but . . . we're at the campground. Victorine and I are together," I said, searching for a way to answer. Was I saying yes? What was I saying?

Lynn looked at me calmly and stroked my hair.

"Come with me back to the ranch. Why don't you both come? Victorine can have a room to herself in the house and you can come stay with me at my cabin up off the north pasture. I'd love to show it to you," he said, looking into my eyes and smiling softly.

I closed my eyes and breathed deeply, collecting my thoughts.

"Do you really want to sleep on that cold ground? I don't want this evening to end," he said.

I opened my eyes, took his face in my hands, kissed him quickly and deliberately and looked into his eyes.

"No, I don't want this evening to end either, but tonight is not the night," I said.

I stood up, reached for his hand and smiled.

"Let's go back inside."

That night, in the tent next to a sleeping Victorine, I lay awake replaying the evening over and over in my mind. I hadn't felt that in a long time, the feeling of being wanted, wanted by someone I wanted. When Victorine awoke in the morning, she found me sitting outside watching the sunrise. She didn't ask any questions. Thankfully, this time she knew when to be silent.

Lynn and Jack met us at the Armadillo Diner for breakfast. They had told us last night that they had a surprise for us today and now they were ready to share their secret.

"We're takin' you ladies to a rodeo," said Lynn, "a real rodeo out near Huntsville. Make sure you bring your camera Victorine 'cause you're gonna want to take some pictures of this. Wait till you see the bull riding."

"Bull riding?" I said.

"Yes, bull riding," said Lynn, "a rider tries to stay on top of a bucking bull for eight seconds."

I was vaguely familiar with what a rodeo was but when I heard this, I told them I wasn't too keen on the idea of going. I was tired from my sleepless night and just wanted to go somewhere where I could relax, maybe alone with Lynn.

"How about we go back to that lake you found and swim?" I suggested.

Victorine would hear none of it. She was adamant that our Texas experience would never be complete without attending a real rodeo. To her, it was the ultimate symbol of the Wild West and during the entire drive she explained to me in minute detail, much to Lynn and Jack's amusement, why I should want to go.

"Listen Natasha, you don't realize but the rodeo began in the middle of the eighteenth century. The cowboys who herded the cattle needed these special skills to earn their living, to survive. First, they had to catch wild horses to ride so they had to learn how to throw a rope and lasso them. The same for calves so they could iron them."

Lynn and Jack both let out a laugh.

"You mean brand them. Cattle are branded with a branding iron," explained Jack, chuckling.

"Yes, yes, exactly," said Victorine, getting more excited. "And once they lassoed the wild horses they had to break them, throw a saddle on them, mount them and stay on without getting bucked off. You see Natasha, it's a celebration of the skills necessary for a cowboy's survival.

We can't go back to New York without having seen a rodeo. Papa would never forgive us if we don't go."

The collected memories of every Wild West movie she had ever seen were playing in her head. She was now in earnest and wanted me to share her enthusiasm.

"Yes, Victorine," I said, "I understand why cowboys needed to ride horses till they stopped bucking and I also understand why it was necessary for cowboys to lasso calves, but please explain to me, when would it ever be necessary for anyone to ride on top of a bull?"

Victorine ignored me and spent the rest of the trip bombarding Lynn and Jack with questions.

Outside the gates of the rodeo arena it looked like a carnival. Everyone seemed in good spirits. Vendors served hot dogs, hamburgers, and cold drinks. A country and western band was playing on a small stage off to the side. There was a booth where you could pay a dollar to try to throw a lasso around a barrel and win a stuffed cow, another where children could get their picture taken atop of a pony.

"Wait here," said Lynn. "We'll be right back with the tickets."

I watched them disappear into the crowd then from behind me heard Victorine exclaim with delight, *"Look, beignets!"*

I turned in time to see her hurrying off towards a food concession stand with a sign above it, "Funnel Cakes." She joined the crowd of people lining up to buy what looked like huge discs of dough the size of dinner plates, deep-fried and covered with powdered sugar.

"Those aren't beignets," I said joining her in line, *"it says,* Funnel Cakes."

"They just look like big Texas-sized beignets to me," she answered, *"Let's share one, I'm hungry."*

When we reached the counter she paid the cashier, selected the largest funnel cake on the tray and held it up for me to taste. I pinched off a piece, tried it, and immediately knew one bite was enough. True, it looked like an enormous beignet but it lacked the delicate consistency of our mother's. This funnel cake was heavy and greasy whereas her beignets were light and puffy. Victorine didn't care. She gobbled up the remainder of our greasy sugary treat then wandered off, disappearing into the crowd just as Lynn and Jack returned with our tickets.

"Where's Victorine?" asked Jack.

"I don't know," I answered.

The three of us craned our necks, scanning the crowd trying to spot her. After a few moments I heard her voice behind me.

"Here, eat this," she said.

I turned around. She was poking something at my face, inches from my nose.

"What's that?" I asked.

"A corn dog," answered Lynn. "It's a hot dog on a stick dipped in corn meal and deep fried."

Victorine took a bite from a half-eaten corn dog she held in her other hand.

"I though you didn't eat meat," said Jack with a confused look.

Victorine ignored his remark and waved the corn dog in my face. I shook my head no.

"Here, try it," she insisted.

"No, I don't want it!" I snapped back.

"I thought she didn't eat meat," Jack said to me, still confused.

Victorine took the last bite from her corn dog, turned to Jack and without a word but with a raise of her eyebrows offered mine to him. He in turn, without a word nodded and accepted it.

Lynn shook his head and said, "We better get inside."

The four of us entered the arena and made our way to our seats in bleachers surrounding a large, enclosed dirt oval. I couldn't help but noticed that in the sea of cowboy hats around us our two escorts were turning quite a few female heads. It wasn't yet noon and the heat was already intense. I squinted up into the bright sunlight.

"Now I know why everyone here wears a cowboy hat," I said. "Frankly I think I could use one with this intolerable heat."

Lynn and Jack exchanged glances then simultaneously removed their hats and gently placed them on our heads. Jack's hat framed Victorine's fine symmetrical features and big dark eyes. She looked gorgeous and I could see in Jack's eyes that he thought so too. He whistled in admiration while Lynn looked at me with a smile. My heart was beating faster. I definitely was falling for him.

"Now you look like cowgirls!" said Jack.

I knew by now, that was the closest these two Texans would come to giving us a compliment.

A voice boomed over the loudspeakers, "Ladies and gentlemen, please welcome today's color guard, our WPRA junior regional champion, Miss Betty-Jo Perkins!"

The crowd burst into wild applause as a beautiful cowgirl atop a magnificent white horse galloped into the arena waving a huge American flag. She circled the edge of the arena then came to a stop in the center.

"Will everyone please stand for our national anthem," the announcer said solemnly. The entire arena rose to its feet, removed their hats and rested their right hands on their hearts as a recording of a military band blared over the loudspeakers. Victorine and I looked at each other and followed suit, a few seconds late. We looked up at Lynn and Jack next to us. They too had their hands over their hearts and were singing with the entire crowd, staring straight at the flag. When the song finished the crowd cheered and sat down.

"Ladies and gentlemen. Are you ready for the timed events?" the announcer roared excitedly into the microphone. "I hope y'all are because you're going to see some amazing events here today: calf roping, barrel racing, bull riding . . ."

The crowd was getting more and more excited, whistling loudly and I heard a few "Yee-Haw's!"

"First on our program is barrel racing. Now don't you go thinkin' barrel racing is easy folks," said the announcer. "It's a timed speed and agility exercise and it can be dangerous, as these ladies know all too well. Now let's give a big welcome to our first rider, Mary Lou Walker from Galveston."

In the middle of the arena were three barrels forming a triangle, each about one hundred feet away from the other. A red-shirted cowgirl astride a beautiful golden palomino exploded through a starting gate at full gallop. She maneuvered her horse, weaving an intricate cloverleaf pattern around the barrels. When she rounded the last one she raced back through the gate at top speed amid cheers and whistles from the crowd.

"Seventeen point five seconds. That's a great time for Mary Lou," the announcer exclaimed.

About ten horses and riders followed. The crowd oohed and aahed in unison as a few of the horses leaned so close to the ground on the turns they looked like they might fall at any moment. I was holding my breath in total admiration of those fearless women who had absolutely no reason to envy the cowboys. These were the real cowgirls of America and their skills were impressive. Lynn turned towards me excitedly and gave me a quick kiss. Jack leaned over to say something to Victorine, who nodded enthusiastically.

I leaned over and said in Victorine's ear, *"You were right, I'm glad we came."*

"Next up is our bull riding competition," the commentator announced excitedly. "As all you Texans know, each rider has to stay atop the bucking bull for eight seconds. It is a risky sport that has been called the most dangerous eight seconds in sports. Let's welcome our first rider, Joe Silverton!"

A cowboy sat mounted on a bull waiting for the gate to open. The huge brown animal bucked furiously inside the small enclosure.

Lynn said softly: "You see, the rider's hand is wrapped around a long braided rope which is attached to the bull. His other hand can't touch the bull. Otherwise he is disqualified."

An air horn blast sounded and suddenly the gate flew open releasing the bull into the arena. He bucked violently while spinning in circles. I held my breath and squeezed Lynn's hand. He clasped mine tighter. After what seemed like an eternity the air horn blasted signaling eight seconds. It seemed to me that the enraged bull was going to buck off its rider every second but the rider held tight. He finally let go and almost gracefully fell to the ground, got up and walked away, all the while keeping a careful eye on the bull who continued to jump and kick.

"Ten point five seconds. Great time!" the commentator announced as the crowd cheered.

"Do you like it?" Lynn asked.

"I don't know, it's scary but it's really interesting," I answered excitedly.

Eight more riders followed suit. Victorine and I were greatly relieved that none of them got hurt even though three riders got bucked off before the eight seconds.

"So this is the surprise, the steer wrestling event," Lynn turned to me and said. "The rider has to jump off his horse onto a steer and wrestle it to the ground by grabbing it by the horns. It's really amazing."

I was skeptical and I was right to be. It was a crazy spectacle. Each cowboy jumped off his galloping horse onto a running steer, grabbed its horns, brutally twisted its neck and wrestling with it until it fell to the ground. To me, it appeared violent and primitive. Wincing, I squeezed Lynn's hand and looked at Victorine. There was a look of utter revulsion on her face. I heard Jack trying to explain to her that it wasn't hurting the steer but she wasn't buying any of it. The crowd's joyful screams were making us feel even more uncomfortable. We excused ourselves and went to get some drinks at the concession stand to avoid the painful sights but the worst was yet to come.

"Next up is our calf-tying event," the commentator announced as we returned.

A young terrified black calf flew out of the gate, while a rider on a white stallion chased it at full speed and launched his lasso in the air. When the lasso fell around the calf's head, the rider yanked it so harshly that the poor calf fell on its back. The rider quickly dismounted his horse and ran to the calf to tie up its three feet. He got up, poker faced, took his horse and walked away while two men ran to untie the calf. My heart sank. I felt like crying. Victorine put her hand over her mouth in horror. We synchronously got up, apologized, and walked back to the concession stand. Jack and Lynn joined us a few minutes later. They both apologized profusely.

"We're really sorry. We had no idea you two were so sensitive," Lynn said.

Neither of us answered. I was about to tell them how brutal and primitive the practice was when I suddenly froze. All at once a memory came to me of a summer holiday I had spent in Madrid with our cousin's family when I was very young. I had gone with them by myself that year because by that time Victorine was old enough to stay home and help our father with the equestrian club. One weekend afternoon our uncle told us we were all going to a *corrida*. I thought it was going to be a fun afternoon outing. I was wearing my favorite little white summer dress and I remember being excited by the sounds and colors when we first entered the arena. Unfortunately it turned out to be one of the most horrible things I ever witnessed.

Maybe I had blocked it out but it all came back to me now. As cruel as this rodeo seemed to me, it didn't reach the degree of horror of the *corridas*, or bullfights, which take place in Spain as well as the south of France. A lone bull is released into an arena and literally slowly tortured to death by six men for the amusement of the applauding spectators. The practice is made even more horrible due to the fact that horses are often killed during these fights. At the start of the spectacle, two *picadors* or men on horseback with lances ride up close to the bull and stab him in order to weaken him. The enraged bull will fight back, charge, often catching them off guard and often goring their horses to death. Once the bull is weakened, three *banderilleros* each take turns stabbing the bull with *banderillas* or barbed sticks that lodge in the bull's flesh, further weakening but enraging him so he will keep fighting. Finally, when the bull is exhausted and weakened from wounds and loss of blood, a single *torero* or chief bullfighter teases the bull a bit more till he is delirious with anger and pain. He then plunges a sword through his back and into his heart, killing him.

Images of that gory afternoon came flooding back to me: the red blood soaking the sandy ground of the arena, the bloodthirsty cheers from the crowd, the hot Spanish sun shining on my little white summer dress which I never wanted to wear again. I remember sitting there horrified yet for some reason stunned and unable to look away. I also remember my mother being so upset when she later found out my uncle brought me to that *corrida* that she didn't talk to him for months.

I was jolted out of my thoughts by Lynn's arm around my shoulder.

"I'm really sorry Natasha," he said softly, "can I make it up to you?"

"No, no. Please just take us back to the campground. We have to get up early tomorrow," I said quietly.

Corn Dogs
Serves 5 to 6

- 1 cup of corn meal
- 2 cups of flour
- 1 lb. of hot dogs
- 1 tablespoon of sugar
- 2 tablespoons of baking powder
- 1 teaspoon of salt
- 2 eggs
- 1 cup of milk
- ¼ cup of oil
- Popsicle sticks

1. In a large bowl mix the milk, eggs, oil, sugar, and salt. Mix it well.
2. Add in the corn meal, flour, and baking powder.
3. Mix it until it is lump free.
4. Dust the hot dogs with flour after having dried them with paper towels.
5. Dip hot dogs into the batter to coat. Dip fry in hot fat and remove when light brown.

Feuilletté au fromage de chèvre
(Puff pastry goat cheese tart)
Serves 2

- 1 large onion, cut into strips
- 4 black figs, halved
- 1 tablespoon of butter
- ¼ cup of pure honey
- 1 tablespoon of brown sugar
- 1 cup of fresh goat cheese, crumbled
- ¼ tablespoon of fresh thyme leaves
- 1 egg, lightly beaten

1. Preheat oven at 400°F.
2. In a small skillet, add the butter, onion, brown sugar, and thyme. Stirring occasionally, cover and sauté the onions until cooked through and caramelized for about 20 to 25 minutes.
3. Unfold the puff pastry on a floured surface and roll out a 10"x 5" sheet. Using a knife, carefully draw a ½" border around the edges of the puff pastry. (Do not cut all the way through the puff pastry).
4. Place the puff pastry on a baking sheet lined with parchment paper and refrigerate for 20 minutes.
5. Remove it from the refrigerator and spread the caramelized onions. Do not go over the ½" border. Refrigerate for another 15 minutes.
6. Sprinkle the goat cheese evenly on the tart over the caramelized onions.
7. Place the halved figs on top.
8. Beat the egg and brush on the edge of the puff pastry.
9. Bake the tart in the center of the oven for 25–30 minutes until the pastry is puffed and golden.
10. Serve hot and sprinkle the tart with honey.

Pâte feuillettée
(Puff Pastry)

- 1 cup of all-purpose flour
- 3 tablespoons of butter, melted
- ½ teaspoon salt
- ½ cup of water
- 10 tablespoons of unsalted butter, cold

Puff pastry has two stages in its fabrication:
- La détrempe
- Le tourage

La détrempe:

1. In a mixing bowl, add flour and make a well.
2. Add the melted butter, salt, and water.
3. Work the mixture well together with hands to form a ball.
4. Refrigerate and let it rest for 2 hours.

Le tourage:

1. Place the dough on a floured surface.
2. Cut a cross on the surface of the dough, then roll out the four corners to form a flattened cross.
3. Shape the cold butter into a square and place it in the middle of dough.
4. Fold the dough over the butter to seal.
5. With a rolling pin, roll gently the entire surface of the dough to make it into a rectangle.
6. Rotate the dough so the "spine" of the fold is on the left. Repeat the rolling and folding.
7. Refrigerate for 30 minutes to 1 hour.
8. Repeat this process over again, refrigerating the dough after you've completed two turns. Then repeat this cycle for a total of 6 turns!
9. Let the dough rest for 1 hour in the fridge before using it.

OR, buy a puff pastry dough in the supermarket!

Chapter Six

Deep in the Heart of a Texan

The interviews with Larry Fitzgerald, LaRoyce Smith, and Farley Matchett were scheduled for the afternoon of our fourth day in Texas. We hadn't slept well, were both feeling rather tense and neither of us were very talkative so rather than waiting in the campground, I suggested we take a drive to calm our nerves. Victorine agreed and as we drove I soon noticed that she was following the signs along the heavily forested area called the "Big Thicket" and heading directly to Terrell Unit. I didn't say a word. Twenty minutes later, we were parked in front of the prison. The sun was bright and it wasn't yet nine a.m. but I felt shrouded in some kind of a mental darkness.

"So this is the place," Victorine murmured gravely, gazing at the somber complex of twenty-three concrete gray buildings sitting amid the lush green Texan landscape. "ALAN B. POLUNSKY UNIT" was written in big white letters on a small concrete rectangular structure. Not wanting to

attract any attention, she discreetly snapped some photos while sitting in the car.

"*I can't believe that after waiting four months this Larry Fitzgerald guy had us come all the way from France to see the death row unit and now that we're here he decides to deny us the visit. What a jerk,*" said Victorine. Her face was contorted as if she had just caught a whiff of something that smelled foul.

"*I'm sure he did it on purpose,*" I said, feeling her fury come over me.

Victorine turned to look at me, her eyes full of anger.

"*That's it. I'm not going to stand for it,*" she said, furiously emphasizing every syllable.

A mischievous grin came over her face.

"*After all, we're just idiots from the European press aren't we?*" she said sarcastically, "*I don't see any reason why we would have understood what he told us on the phone. We thought that we were going to visit the death row unit this morning at 9 a.m., right?*"

I smiled slyly.

"*Quite right,*" I agreed.

Victorine reached behind her head, removed the elastic band holding her ponytail and shook out her long brown hair. She pulled her lipstick out of her purse and applied it looking in the rear view mirror. She then pinched some color into her cheeks, undid one more button on her blouse, quickly stepped out of the car, and walked purposefully towards the metal barracks on our right. Although a bit scared and not knowing exactly what to expect, I followed behind. A tall guard with a moustache looked up from his desk and flashed us a big yellow-toothed smile as we neared the gate.

"Howdy! My name is Victorine and this is Natasha. We're reporters scheduled to visit the prison this morning to interview some inmates," Victorine said with a tone of voice that could have melted butter.

"Well, good morning ladies," the guard said as he slowly looked us up and down. "Let me check with the warden."

He picked up a phone and made a call.

"Yes, I've got two reporters here. They say they're scheduled to visit the prison this morning and interview some inmates," he said into the receiver. "Uh huh . . . Uh huh . . . okay."

He hung up the phone and turned to look at us.

"Wait right here," he said. "The warden is on his way. So, you certainly have a lovely accent. Let me guess . . . German?"

I was surprised to hear Victorine let out a giggly schoolgirl laugh, totally out of her character.

"No silly," she said, "we're from France."

We endured a few minutes of inane chitchat with the tall guard then another man showed up at the door. He looked at us quizzically. Victorine kept the same charming smile pasted on her face while I stood silent and stiff as a mummy.

"Good morning, I'm Warden Phillips," he said. Then flipping through the pages on his clipboard he continued, "Vick-ter-reen and Natasha Saulnier, well, I have you scheduled for an interview this afternoon with two inmates, but . . ."

"Well, actually, we talked to Larry Fitzgerald yesterday evening. Maybe he was in a rush to get home and forgot to call you. He definitely said we should come this morning at nine a.m.," Victorine said confidently.

Terrified, I nervously flashed my plastic laminated New York press pass and nodded with an innocent smile. My heart was pounding. I knew that if Larry Fitzgerald found out we were defying his orders he would forbid us from interviewing Farley Matchett and LaRoyce Smith now and forever. I was expecting him to say he was going to check with Larry, but instead he looked us up and down and said quietly, "Well, ladies, you have to excuse Larry, you know, with all these prisoners he has a hard time keeping up with the media. I'll have to remind you though, no cameras allowed inside."

Victorine nodded and answered in a sweet voice, "Oh, we totally understand," then abracadabra, open sesame! There was a loud buzz and the heavy white gate swung open to let us in. I was so excited that I had to turn around to compose myself.

"Follow me, ladies," the warden instructed.

He led us down a hallway through a series of heavy blue metal gates that slammed shut loudly behind us as we passed through each one.

"These gates separate the population into small units in case there is a riot," he said, "You can see here, ladies, we never open two gates at the same time."

As a gate closed behind me I looked up and saw a sign printed in blue on one of the white walls. Some ominous words, calling to mind a fraternity's code of silence, it read:

"LOYALTY: IF YOU WORK FOR TDCJ, IN HEAVEN'S NAME WORK FOR THIS INSTITUTION. SPEAK WELL OF THE INSTITUTION AND STAND BY THE INSTITUTION YOU REPRESENT. REMEMBER AN OUNCE OF LOYALTY IS WORTH A POUND OF CLEVERNESS. IF YOU MUST GROWL, CONDEMN AND ETERNALLY FIND FAULT, RESIGN YOUR POSITION. BUT AS LONG AS YOU ARE PART OF THIS INSTITUTION, DO NOT CONDEMN IT. IF YOU DO, THE FIRST HIGH WIND THAT COMES ALONG WILL BLOW YOU AWAY AND PROBABLY YOU WILL NEVER KNOW WHY."

We followed him through a fenced hallway past the inquisitive gaze of the general population's inmates, all dressed in white uniforms. I was surprised that we heard no whistles or catcalls from them as we passed. A skinny dark-haired guard in a grey uniform standing at the next gate eyed us curiously as we approached.

"This is Lieutenant Roach, he supervises the death row unit," the warden said, his hand resting on the man's shoulder. "He is going to take over from here. Unfortunately I can't continue your tour. I have some business to attend to. Goodbye ladies."

Lieutenant Roach seemed to enjoy the attention and welcomed our presence in the sinister environment. He smiled at us and invited us to follow him as he briskly walked down the hall. We passed through another massive blue metal gate and it closed behind us with another thunderous slam. A sign overhead read, "Building number 12." I held my breath. Despite all odds, we had made it into the death row unit where about four hundred inmates were locked up in single-person cells.

I found myself growing more and more claustrophobic as we spent the next hour that seemed like an eternity passing through one locked iron gate after another. The atmosphere was unbelievable oppressive, much worse than I had ever imagined. I followed closely behind Lieutenant Roach and frantically scribbling in my notebook, forcing myself to breathe deeply through my mouth to keep from passing out. We finally exited through the main gate into sunshine and walked back toward the parking lot.

"*We did it, we did it*," sang Victorine as she jumped up and down in a little victory dance. I ran to the nearest tree and vomited up my breakfast.

"Are you all right?" I heard a voice ask from behind.

I turned around and saw an elegant blonde woman who I judged to be in her mid-fifties standing over me, looking genuinely concerned.

"We just visited the death row unit, she'll be okay in a moment." answered Victorine, stepping protectively between us, handing me a tissue.

The woman gave me a moment to compose myself. Thankfully my nausea was starting to fade now that my breakfast was on the ground.

"Are you journalists?" she asked.

"Yes," answered Victorine.

"My husband is the prison chaplain. I shouldn't really be speaking to you . . ." she began but her words trailed off. This woman clearly had something to say but was struggling to keep her words contained. I took a step closer.

"Please go on," I said softly.

She hesitated then continued.

". . . but this is a very sad place. Most of these inmates are totally abandoned. They have no family visits until the day before their execution and they are deprived of more and more privileges each . . ."

The woman's body stiffened and her eyes widened. I looked over my shoulder to follow the direction of her gaze and noticed a large dark sedan exiting the parking lot. The uniformed driver's head turned toward us as he slowly rolled up to the stop sign. He sat there motionless, his arm resting on the window ledge, the sun reflecting off his dark sunglasses. The only sound was the idling of the car's engine. After an uncomfortable moment he drove off slowly. The woman quickly wished us good luck with our story and nervously departed.

In a flash the words written in blue on the white wall, the code of silence, the "Loyalty Oath" became crystal clear to me. Those concrete and razor wire walls built to hold the inmates were tangible, but almost as suffocating were the invisible walls that held the prison employees' souls. Obviously, if this "Loyalty Oath" was printed on the wall, there had been past problems with employees voicing their opinions to the outside world. Although we were outside in the bright Texas sunshine, I suddenly felt claustrophobic and my nausea returned.

"*OK. I think we've seen and heard enough for a while,*" said Victorine. "*Let's get the hell out of here. I know where we can go to go to relax before the interviews.*"

Back on the highway we drove in silence. I genuinely think that Victorine was shocked by what we had seen but pragmatic as usual, she was keeping a cool head. I knew she wanted to talk about our uncommon experience but she knew I needed some time to escape that abominable place, and process all I had seen in my own time. Thankfully, she respected my silence. We drove out to a nearby lake where I sat quietly in the grass while she studiously observed and photographed some insects, frogs, and turtles along the shoreline. My stomach slowly became quiet.

At 2:00 p.m. we returned to the prison to meet with Larry Fitzgerald, who thankfully hadn't yet gotten wind of our morning excursion in the death row unit. He took us to the visiting parlor where the interviews were scheduled to take place. Farley Matchett sat waiting patiently in a booth behind a thick wall of glass, his hands crossed on the table. A telephone handset hung on the wall to my left. Larry Fitzgerald sat behind us while two female guards closely monitored our every word and move.

I lifted the handset. Farley Matchett, a handsome, self-possessed thirty-eight-year-old black man greeted me on the other end and told me it was nice to finally meet in person after years of exchanging letters. I knew from his letters that he was a very intelligent, articulate, and determined man. The story he told, describing a blatant mockery of justice, was particularly compelling. Larry Fitzgerald's presence made me uncomfortable and I immediately asked Farley to tell us his story. Victorine took some photos of him then sat down next to me. "I'll take some more when you're done with your story," she said.

"My story is a tragic one of misfortune, duplicity, and racism," he began in a very collected voice. It was difficult to concentrate on his words let alone hear him because the guards were speaking loudly and making jokes behind me.

"On July eleventh nineteen ninety one, I engaged in a conversation with a man to whom I had loaned money. After I asked him when he was going to settle his eight-month old debt, he became angry so I tried to leave, but when I did he struck me with his fist. We fought but he was much bigger than me. He grabbed a knife and tried to slash my throat. I pushed the knife back towards him. It lodged in his chest and he immediately fell. I called the paramedics but he died in surgery later. Three days later, I was arrested and interrogated for thirty-six brutal hours during which the detectives literally beat a confession out of me. I couldn't see the paper because of my swollen eyes, so the detective led my hand in signing the confession. I was then thrown into an underground cell for nineteen long months to await my trial. The trial began on February twenty second, nineteen ninety-three. It was over February twenty sixth, nineteen ninety-three. My court-appointed lawyer told me to plead guilty to avoid a death sentence. He said he would introduce the self-defense plea later. I complied because I trusted him but in fact, he set me up to get the death sentence. He called only two witnesses during the punishment phase. He made no objections and in nineteen ninety-six, the appeals courts turned me down on my first appeal because of this. They stated that the lawyer failed to enter a noted objection and since he didn't, they couldn't enter it for him. If he had, they would have granted me a new trial."

Farley had been calm and collected at the start of the interview but as his story progressed his voice and mannerisms became more and more animated. His speech was getting louder and louder and his eyes grew wide with an eerie unfocused intensity. I thought about all the time he had spent alone in isolation anticipating our arrival and realized he must have rehearsed his soliloquy repeatedly for just this moment. He continued.

"My victim was portrayed as a white man married to a black woman before a jury of eleven whites and one black. Years later, a lawyer investigating the case reviewed an autopsy report and noted that the victim's race was listed as black. His features looked more white than black but legally he was black. If they had portrayed the victim as black, I wouldn't be sitting here on death row or in any other jail. In Texas, executions are so common that they no longer make the front page of the Huntsville newspaper. Governor Bush has stood over one hundred forty five executions in five years he's been in office. He has vetoed bills that would stop the execution of the mentally retarded or mentally ill. There is no justice for the poor, the mentally retarded, the mentally ill, and people of color . . ."

The long-winded speech was obviously getting too militant for Larry Fitzgerald, who got up and announced that the interview was over.

"But it only lasted a quarter of an hour," I argued.

"And I haven't had a chance to take good photos of him," Victorine added.

"Take a few shots and say goodbye to him. It's time for the next visit," snapped Larry Fitzgerald.

Farley looked at us and in his eyes I heard a silent prayer he had no need to articulate. Deeply disturbed by his story and by its interruption, we watched as he was led away by the guards. We heard the now familiar sound of a slamming iron gate, the jingling of keys turning in a lock, and watched as LaRoyce Smith was led in and seated in the same chair behind the thick glass. A strongly built black man with a cherubic face and glasses, LaRoyce welcomed us with a sweet smile. At thirty-one years old he had a mixed aura of childish candor and dignity. He picked up his handset.

"Hello LaRoyce. It's nice to meet you."

"Hello, Natasha, it's nice to meet you at last."

LaRoyce spoke very slowly and his English was ungrammatical. He had a gentle smile on his face and honestly, despite his age, he looked as if he was nineteen years old, which is precisely the age he was when he was convicted to death. His entire demeanor stood in sharp contrast to Farley's. Victorine stood up and began taking photos. I sensed Larry Fitzgerald leaning closer to hear what I said.

"Unfortunately we don't have much time, LaRoyce, so why don't you tell us your story?"

Victorine took a few more photos then sat next to me to listen. LaRoyce began speaking slowly and calmly. I had found LaRoyce's letters particularly moving because in them he described a dreamlike universe where he would retreat to escape the dehumanizing environment of death row. He wrote that he would often imagine himself flying in the sky with the birds, which he managed to catch sight of standing up on the bunk in his cell. This was the first time he had spoken with reporters and I found it interesting how composed and dignified he appeared. As I listened to him speak, it became clear that he hadn't reached his full mental maturity.

"Well, on January ninth, nineteen ninety-one, I was nineteen years old then, me and my four friends are drivin' around, just drivin' around and the next thing I know we parked behind a Taco Bell. Kevin, Kevin Shaw says, 'I'm gonna hit Taco Bell tonight.' Ya see, Travis, Travis Brown was working there with the closing manager, Jennifer, Jennifer Soto. Well Kevin says, "It's all set, Travis is leavin' the back door open. He jumps out the car and goes to the back door and pulls on it. Well, the three of us is jus' waitin' in the car but Travis don't come out."

LaRoyce hesitated as he glanced over my shoulder at Larry Fitzgerald who I could tell was listening intently.

"Yes go on," I said, glancing over my shoulder.

"Well, like I said, Travis don't come out," he continued, "so we drive away, but Kevin get all mad and says, 'we goin' back.' We pull 'round back and Kevin gets out an' knocks on the back door. Travis opens it now, and Kevin, Devario, and me goes in. I don't see Jennifer nowhere and stay in back with Travis and everybody else and Kevin goes up front to the office. Then, I hear a BANG and I run to the office. Kevin's hittin' Jennifer with a gun. The gun broke and Kevin tells Jennifer to open the safe. She just sits there and he screams, 'Open the safe, bitch,' but she say she don't know the combination. Kevin runs to the kitchen and grabs up a butcher knife and starts stabbing Jennifer. I'm thinkin' oh no, oh no, what's this? . . . 'cause you see I knew Jennifer and liked her. I grabbed the bloody knife away from Kevin and I run out the back door with it but Kevin was out there already and told

Leabharlanna Poiblí Chathair Bhaile Átha Cliath
Dublin City Public Libraries

everybody I killed Jennifer. Travis said, 'Damn, man, that wasn't even in it,' like that killing Jennifer was not part of the plan. I'm thinkin'... Plan? What plan? I didn't know nothin' about no plan. Later my so-called friends who hadn't even seen what happened all testified against me. Only Kevin Shaw was convicted to a prison sentence but I was convicted of capital murder."

"What happened during the trial?" Victorine asked softly.

LaRoyce took a deep breath and exhaled slowly.

"Well, they found a witness who signed a statement sayin' he heard Kevin boastin' about the murder and that he escaped capital punishment and all but my first lawyer didn't ask him to testify. I found out later that he never handled a capital murder case before. He didn't even tell the judge that I never been violent in the past. Then my other lawyer let the deadline pass to submit a appeal..."

After listening to Farley's story and now LaRoyce's I felt like my head was spinning. Victorine and I were both speechless. Of course, we do not presume to know the truth about really what happened during those ill-fated days Farley and LaRoyce's lives drifted uncontrollably, we are not deluded about human nature—still it was hard to listen to LaRoyce without having the feeling that one was dealing with a child. The justice system's malfunctions, as described by those two inmates, seemed simply shocking. LaRoyce looked down at his hands, took another deep breath and continued.

"Look, I am not askin' to be let out. I know I deserve to be punished for being involved the robbery but I don't deserve to be killed. I agree to spend another five years in jail but I don't wanna die. I want another trial to tell the world my version of what happened and hold my son in my arms..."

Fitzgerald suddenly announced that the interview was over. I was about to protest that we needed more time but LaRoyce just smiled. He knew he had to comply. I was at a loss for words but quickly blurted out, "We will do our best to tell your version of the story to the world, LaRoyce. We will write to you. Goodbye."

"Goodbye, Natasha. Thank you with all my heart for coming to see me and listening to my story," he said softly.

On January 17, 2007, thanks to Amnesty International, the US Supreme Court commuted LaRoyce's sentence to life in prison based on the decision that the jurors had not been directed to consider mitigating circumstances of childhood abuse and limited mental capacity. LaRoyce managed to escape the maddening universe of death row, after all.

Despite the pleas to Governor Rick Perry by *And God Created Women* star Brigitte Bardot, who said she would help pay Farley's legal fees if he was given another trial, Farley Matchett, prisoner number 999060, was executed on September 12, 2006, in front of the victim's family. He was put to death by lethal injection and pronounced dead at 6:16 p.m.

I am aware that the touching story Farley told us differs greatly from the official one. He never revealed to me nor his French supporters that he was a crack addict. He mentioned that the victim had a chest wound but the autopsy refers to back and head wounds. His story about the paramedics also appeared to be false. After researching a number of legal documents, I ended up believing LaRoyce's story but I suspect Farley was lying despite his appearance of utter sincerity. Why did Farley manipulate so many people when he obviously knew the legal documents condemned him? Was he a mythomaniac? Did he suffer from a personality disorder, stemming from his horrible childhood, which compelled him to manipulate people? I am now more convinced than ever, thanks to LaRoyce's story, that the court-appointed lawyers who defend those inmates are often the worst-paid, most inexperienced, and least skillful lawyers. Indeed, how could somebody like LaRoyce end up on death row? Farley is a different story. Unfortunately Farley's probable lies did a huge disservice to the abolitionist movement. As I said before, the death penalty is a very complicated issue but I am convinced that "an eye for an eye" is not a way to heal our world.

Something else really irks me. Like many aspects of our cultural shocks in America, it had to do with food. During my research I came across a book entitled *Meals to Die For* published in 2004 and written by "death row chef" Brian Price. It presents inmates' bios, their crimes, describes their last meals, and lists morbid "jailhouse" recipes such as "Old Sparky's Genuine Convict Chili," "Post Mortem Potato Soup," and "Hangman's Spaghetti." At first glance, it sheds a disturbing light on some people's ghoulish fascination with death and paradoxically points to the inmates' humanity. "One man ordered butter beans, which was difficult to prepare, but it was something his mum made him when he was a kid and I knew it would take him back to a time when it was peaceful," wrote Price in an article published in the *Observer*. However, more than anything it highlighted an unhealthy relationship with food. To me, the association of a vital agent like food with death or murder is simply shocking.

For his last meal, Farley Matchett requested four olives and a bottle of wild berry flavored water.

As difficult as the day had been, I was more ill-prepared for what was to happen next. We were scheduled to fly back to New York the next day and had plans to spend the evening with Jack and Lynn to say goodbye. After going back to the campground to freshen up, we joined them at the Longhorn BBQ near Huntsville hoping to spend a relaxing evening and forget our difficult day. Jack and Lynn were dressed in the same black outfits they wore the first night we went out with them but perhaps due to my mental exhaustion, tonight his good looks didn't have the same effect on me. Both men seemed to be in an excellent mood as they led us to a table near the back of the crowded restaurant, which consisted of two long rows of picnic tables lined up along walls hung with mounted steer heads. The configuration of the tables and the décor created the effect of an outdoor barbecue transported indoors. The floor was covered with a layer of sawdust and peanut shells, music blared from a large old-fashioned neon-lit jukebox near the front door, and vented open grills covered with rows of searing meat lined the rear wall.

"I know the menu at this place like the back of my hand. It has the best down home barbecue in the county," said Lynn. "Let me order a few plates of ribs for the table. You're gonna love it."

He waved to an attractive middle-aged blond waitress who obediently sashayed over to our table.

"Hello there darlin'," he said as she neared.

I looked up just in time to see him give her a wink as she pulled her order book from her back pocket and a pencil from behind her ear.

"Well, well, if it isn't Mister Lynn Elmwood," she said, "Haven't seen you in a dog's age. Looks like you and your friend here have been keepin' yourselves busy."

She looked at Victorine and me then back to Lynn and gave him a wink and a little laugh.

"Come on darlin', you know I can't stay away from your barbecue for long. Why don't you bring us two orders of your house special and a round of beers," said Lynn.

Victorine must have been just as tired as me because neither of us protested when two huge platters of barbecued ribs, enough to feed two families, arrived at the table. I took sip from the bottle of beer placed in front of me and listened with half an ear while Lynn and Jack sang the praises of local barbecue sauces and argued over which roadside stand had the most authentic flavor. I wasn't in the mood for small talk and the loud music and raucous conversations from the adjoining tables was starting to give me a headache. My nerves were on edge after our traumatic day and I was eager to vent some of my pent up emotions. I decided to introduce the issue that was gnawing at me.

"So today, we actually visited the death row unit. It was quite an ordeal. A necessary ordeal though," I announced sighing heavily, looking directly at Lynn to watch his reaction. Victorine reached toward one of the platters, grabbed a large rib, and began gnawing on it. After eight years as a vegetarian she was eating corn dogs and now beef ribs? The sight triggered a strange feeling inside me and I began to feel very odd.

"Wait a minute, I thought TDCJ didn't wanna to let you in," said Jack.

"Well . . . we convinced the warden and a guard gave us a tour," said Victorine with a sly smile. "But wow, it was just like a science-fiction movie in there. You wouldn't believe how they treat those poor guys."

The two men looked at each other, raised their bottles, and drained their beers. Their faces changed and darkness came over them, different from the good-natured men we were used to.

"Well, what did you expect? They're murderers in there. Those guys are dirt . . . scum," said Lynn with a look of disgust.

"Well yes, some are murderers, of course, but some might be innocent," I answered.

"Oh come on, wake up. If those guys were innocent they wouldn't be in there," said Lynn, his voice getting louder.

"Oh, yes, that's right. Each and every one of them are super predators," I said sarcastically.

"Damn right, they are!" said Jack, banging his fist on the table, causing a few empty beer bottles to topple and both Victorine and me to jump.

Both men were now on their third beer but they had probably started drinking before meeting us and the alcohol was now disinhibiting them. Their voices were getting louder, they were getting more and more passionate, and I realized that all this time they had probably been holding back from confronting us on this issue. Their eyes were wide and they were getting worked up. I lost my appetite as I watched the pile of gnawed bones pile up on the table.

"Seriously, have you ever heard of the Innocence Project?" asked Victorine. "Are you aware that DNA evidence has exonerated approximately fourteen people on death row in the United States? Do you think they should have been killed?"

"Hey, I say execute them right away rather than waste years of honest taxpayer's money feedin' them," said Jack, ignoring Victorine's question, "I'll tell you, there's a reason why almost all the criminals in prison are black . . . crime is in their blood."

"Damn straight," said Lynn.

I felt like I had been punched in the stomach. I was furious but held my tongue. I looked at Victorine who was sitting with her mouth open in disbelief. She had the expression of someone who has come across a nasty snake during a beautiful walk. My head began to throb. I pushed my plate away and breathed deeply. It would take a wealth of patience to educate those two Texans on some very essential truths about democratic societies' justice systems.

"The only problem with Texas is that we're too lax with criminals," Lynn said loudly.

I laughed loudly. Victorine pushed her plate that was covered with rib bones away with a look of disgust on her face. The men had finished eating and now were just drinking beer. The empty bottles lined up on the table were starting to make me more and more uncomfortable.

"Let me tell you, back in my grandpa's day they knew how to handle criminals," said Lynn leaning back in his chair. "None of this liberal justice system, let me tell you." He spat out the words "liberal justice" as if they tasted bad on his tongue. "If a man was caught stealing another man's cattle or touching another man's wife or daughter, they'd find the nearest tree and have a neck tie party right then and there."

"Damn straight," added Jack. "Prairie justice saves a lot of time and money."

Both Victorine and I blinked in disbelief.

"What do you mean by 'neck tie party' and 'prairie justice'?" I asked.

Both men laughed even more raucously and all eyes turned to look at us. The whole scene was really starting to get pathetic and we were right in the middle of it.

"What do you mean?" I demanded.

I didn't need to ask. I knew the answer but wanted to hear them say it. My previous image of two well-bred Texans evaporated before my eyes. Deep in the heart of my Texan was a narrow-minded racist I had absolutely no desire to associate with.

"*Well, I guess, in vino veritas,*" said Victorine as she threw some money on the table. "*The beer has loosened their tongues and finally we learn the truth about who they really are.*"

"*There's no point trying to explain anything to them,*" I said bitterly as I rose, reaching for my bag.

"Well, sirs, it's really been a pleasure but it's late and we've had a hard day . . ." Victorine said to the two disconcerted men. She stood up quickly, turned to leave, then whirled back and looked at them both with disgust on her face.

" . . . and one more thing. Life isn't as easy for everyone as it is for you two. Not everyone inherits oil wells and can get a job by simply snapping their fingers, and you," she said pointing to Lynn, "Not everyone's lucky enough to have a daddy who can buy him ponies so he can ride around and play cowboy."

"*Come on, let's get out of here before I get really upset,*" she muttered.

The only sound was the honky-tonk music from the jukebox and every head turned to watch Victorine storm out of the restaurant. I followed without looking back. Well, I suppose disappointment can accompany enlightenment, I thought. In the car, I was feeling like an idiot and didn't want to think about Lynn's betrayal too long.

"*I'm glad that happened when it did. You were falling for him,*" said Victorine.

"*I think I was. He was really handsome and he seemed so nice at first,*" I said, feeling my heart in my throat.

"*Well you're not the first woman to fall for the wrong guy,*" she said softly.

During the flight back to New York thoughts and images swirled in my head: those of Lynn of course, but also Victor Hugo's short novel *The Last Day of a Condemned Man* and my favorite writer Albert Camus' stance on the death penalty. The fiasco with Lynn seemed to prevent me from organizing my thoughts and I was struggling to remember one of Camus' quotes on the death penalty. Totally discouraged, I burst into tears. I needed time to process my experience with Lynn quietly on my own. Suddenly I remembered the quote. I found a pen in my purse and scribbled it down on the back of an airsick bag I found in the seat pocket in front of me.

"*Capital punishment is the most premeditated of murders, to which no criminal's deed, however calculated can be compared. For there to be an equivalency, the death penalty would have to punish a criminal who had warned his victim of the date at which he would inflict a horrible death on him and who, from that moment onward, had confined him at his mercy for months. Such a monster is not encountered in private life.*"

Texas Longhorn BBQ Ribs
Serves 4

- 2 slabs pork spareribs
- ½ cup of tomato base
- 2 cups of water
- 2 teaspoons vegetable oil
- 2 tablespoon of honey
- 3 tablespoon of Worcestershire sauce
- ¼ cup minced fresh onion
- 1 tablespoon minced garlic
- 3 tablespoons paprika
- 1 tablespoon dried thyme
- 1 tablespoon chili powder
- 2 tablespoons of whiskey
- ¼ teaspoon of freshly ground pepper
- ¼ teaspoon of salt

1. For the barbecue sauce, heat oil in large saucepan over medium heat. Add chopped onion and garlic and cook 4 to 5 minutes until lightly browned.
2. Stir in the tomato base, water, Worcestershire sauce, paprika, thyme, chili powder, and the whiskey.
3. Add honey, salt, and pepper and bring it to a boil.
4. Reduce heat and simmer stirring occasionally for 10 minutes.
5. Heat grill. Place in center of grill. Cover and grill ribs over low heat 275°F to 300°F for 1½ hours, adding 5 to 10 briquettes to each side every 20 minutes (if using a charcoal grill).
6. Put aside 1 cup of barbecue sauce for basting. During last hour of cooking, brush ribs with some of the basting sauce every 10 to 15 minutes until meat is very tender.
7. Serve ribs with remaining sauce.

Andouillettes au Vin Blanc
(Andouillette with White Wine)
Serves 4

- 4 Andouillettes
- 1 bay leaf
- 1 sprig of thyme
- 4 shallots
- 4 tablespoons of grain mustard
- 1 large glass of white wine
- 1 tablespoon of butter
- Salt and pepper to taste

1. Heat the oven to 350°F.
2. Peel and cut the shallots finely and place them in an oven-proof dish with the thyme and bay leaf. Pour over the wine.
3. Bake in the oven for 20-30 minutes.
4. Put the andouillettes aside. Place the sauce in a saucepan with the butter and mustard.
5. Pour the sauce over the andouillettes on a plate.
6. Can be served with French fries or mashed potatoes.

Chapter Seven

Serpentine Salvation

We returned to our apartment in Queens where I finished writing and editing our story. Victorine proofed and selected her photos and we submitted our article. The trip had lasted less than a week but it felt as if I had returned from a long, arduous journey. We spent the next few weeks exploring the city, searching out interesting ideas for new magazine articles. We interviewed female private investigators for a story on "The Real Charlie's Angels" and a fluff piece on department store mannequins and what they say about ourselves, but all the while we were excitedly preparing for our next big out of town reportage about rural religious fundamentalism. We were going to meet the "snake handlers" of the Pentecostal Church of Lord Jesus in Jolo, West Virginia. Jolo is a little town in Appalachia, or "God's country" as its inhabitants sometimes call it. Snake handlers are believers who interpret certain passages in the King James Bible literally:

And these signs shall follow them that believe: In my name shall they cast out devils; they shall speak with new tongues. They shall take up serpents; and if they drink any deadly thing, it shall not hurt them; they shall lay hands on the sick, and they shall recover. (Mark 16:17–18)

Behold, I give unto you power to tread on serpents and scorpions, and over all the power of the enemy: and nothing shall by any means hurt you. (Luke 10:19)

The practice originated in southeastern Tennessee as an offshoot of the Pentecostal Holiness movement spreading through backwoods Appalachia in the first half of the twentieth century. Serpent handling is illegal in every state of the Union, except West Virginia where the members of the congregation feel free to talk to the media. During our phone conversation, Reverend Elkins, whose family had founded the Church of Jolo, was very welcoming. He told me that since there was neither hotel nor campground in the vicinity of the church, he would arrange for us to sleep at the home of one the congregants "who had already accommodated journalists." The thought of sleeping in the house of snake-handlers made me a bit apprehensive but I contacted some Swedish reporters who had stayed there the year before and they reassured me it was safe.

It was early October but the air was still warm in New York City. The summer had been very humid and we were looking forward to cooling down while exploring the Appalachian Mountains. We picked up the rental car in the afternoon, and after a preparatory nap and a quick stop to fill our thermos with Dunkin' Donuts coffee to brace ourselves for the twelve-hour drive, we were on the road by midnight. Highway driving is always smoother at night. I pulled out our little carrying case of travel CDs and in the company of Dalida, the French singer of old romantic French melodies, as well as other singers of "chansons françaises" like Charles Aznavour and Gilbert Bécaud, the hours ticked by pleasantly. Around sunrise we spotted a sign for a rest stop near Greenville, Virginia.

"*I'm starving. Let's stop and get breakfast,*" said Victorine, swerving quickly from the left lane across the morning commuter traffic toward the exit. Although a safe driver, Victorine's confidence behind the wheel could be occasionally disconcerting when zipping through gaps between speeding cars that I'd have gauged too small if I were behind the wheel. I had no choice. She always insisted upon doing all the driving, never relinquishing control.

We stretched our legs as we walked across the huge parking lot filled with massive idling trucks lined up in neat rows. Yellow and red lights outlined their exteriors and the bright overhead lights of the parking lot reflecting off the shining chrome and mirrors in the still dim early morning reminded me of a carnival. Inside, we found two seats at the counter of the brightly lit chrome-trimmed diner. On either side of us sat bleary-eyed truckers hunched over steaming mugs of coffee. Victorine snatched up a menu and scanned it. I did the same and instantly became hungry as I looked at the pages and pages of food choices.

"Look at this," I said pointing to the menu, "French toast, I wonder what that is?"

"I don't know," answered Victorine pointing to her menu, "but I'm getting this, sausage, eggs, and grits."

Starting on that last day in Texas when she had devoured a plate of barbeque ribs, Victorine had inexplicably abandoned her vegetarianism. Now here she was sitting in front of me eating a huge helping of eggs, grits, toast and the most greasy, unappetizing sausages I had ever seen.

"Are those good?" I asked doubtfully.

Victorine didn't answer. She just nodded and continued eating. I looked down at my plate. My French toast turned out to be nothing more than egg-soaked bread, fried and covered with butter and powdered sugar. It was unbearably sweet, too sweet for breakfast. I ate a few bites then pushed my plate away, sat back, and drank my third cup of coffee.

When we reached the majestic George Washington National Forest in Virginia, I rolled down the window and breathed in the crisp mountain air and the fresh smell of the tall pine trees. Victorine, who always had a knack for creating an unforgettable musical ambiance, popped in a CD and played John Denver's "Take Me Home, Country Roads." The car was quickly filled with our off-key yet enthusiastic singing.

"Country roads, take me home to the place I belong, West Virginia, mountain mama, take me home, country roads . . ."

Yes, West Virginia was almost heaven with its green lush vegetation and its strangely soothing mountains. Chipmunks and squirrels occasionally darted across the road and Victorine braked quickly, causing the tires to screech loudly and us to laugh hysterically. Different species of songbirds such as the Mourning Dove, the Northern Cardinal, and Blue Jay flew in front of our car and we felt strangely free. At one point we even saw what had to be a Bald Eagle circling high overhead. It was impossible not to stop along the way to photograph old barns or abandoned cars and even cows grazing in the fields, but when we reached McDowell County on Route 83, we realized that we had really left civilization behind. Unfortunately, it also meant that poverty was overwhelmingly rampant and showed itself with its ramshackle houses, dilapidated mobile homes, and junk piled around abandoned houses and barns nestled in the depths of the green mountains. There was no flat ground, only towering hills and vertiginous hollows. The combination of dramatic landscape and the blatant poverty was a bit overwhelming.

McDowell County, formerly famous for its coal mining industry, used to be a major player in the state's economy. There were testimonies of it everywhere: abandoned railroad loading stations, empty dilapidated factories, scarred and blasted hillsides, but the industry began to decline in the 1950s and younger residents moved out of the county to seek better futures, leaving behind an older and increasingly impoverished population. In the 1980s, the county went from painful decline to heartbreaking collapse as the steel production in the United States declined due to foreign competition. No county in the Appalachian region was more severely distressed by these losses than McDowell County and by the 1990s the poverty rate in McDowell County was 37.7 percent, the highest rate of poverty for any county in West Virginia. By 1990, 50.3 percent of all children in McDowell County were living in homes below the poverty level. Many walked away from their mortgages and simply abandoned their homes to the lenders.

"*Let's stop for some food,*" said Victorine, "*I haven't eaten for hours and I'm starting to feel weak.*"

"*It's five o'clock now!*" I cried, "*We don't have time. We have to be there in half an hour.*"

"*But I have to eat,*" moaned Victorine.

"*We're late and it's your fault,*" I said, "*you kept stopping to take your photos.*"

"*I don't care,*" she said, "*look, a McDonald's. We're stopping here.*"

I continued to protest but Victorine ignored me, pulled into the parking lot and slowed the car as she peered intently through the windshield. I followed her gaze to a yellow sign, "Drive Thru Lane." She slowly pulled ahead and stopped next to a huge outdoor menu surrounded by colorful photos of each item listed.

"Welcome to McDonald's, kin I take your order," asked a cheery, disembodied female voice.

Victorine looked at me with a huge grin then back towards the menu.

"Yes you can," she answered, "I'd like a hamburger, large French fries and a Coke."

"Okay, would ya like anything else?"

Victorine looked over at me. Fuming I sat with my arms folded, staring straight ahead as I shook my head. She turned back to the menu and addressed the disembodied voice.

"Yes, another large French fries and a Coke."

"Okay, that'll be five sixty three. You kin pick up your order at window two."

We slowly drove forward and stopped next to the second window. A young red-haired woman wearing a headset with microphone and baseball cap with a McDonald's logo poked her head out the window, took our money, handed Victorine a bag then disappeared back inside as she spoke into her headset, "Welcome to McDonald's, kin I take your order."

Victorine quickly peered inside the bag, handed it to me with a self-satisfied grin then pulled out of the parking lot and back out onto the road.

"There," she said, *"It took no time at all, now hand me my burger."*

We ate in silence as we drove. Victorine had one hand on the steering wheel while she happily held her burger with the other. This was our first stop at a drive thru restaurant . . . it wouldn't be our last.

When we finally reached Jolo at 5:30 p.m. it appeared deserted, like a ghost town with nothing but a gas station, a little grocery store, a honky-tonk, and a post office. We asked for directions from two tousle-haired teenagers who were tinkering with an old motorbike in front of the gas station. The Church of Lord Jesus turned out to be a small modest white wooden house sitting on the edge of a deep ravine just up the road. As we pulled into the parking lot we saw a gray-haired man with glasses unloading two long flat boxes from the back of his pickup truck.

"Hello, my name is Natasha and this is Victorine. We're looking for Reverend Elkins," I said to him.

"Well, hello. God welcomes you here with us today. I'm Reverend Elkins," he answered, "You must be the reporters from France I spoke with on the phone. Come inside, please. You're just in time for the 7 p.m. service."

We followed him though the front double doors into a large single room with eight rows of green upholstered pews on either side of a central aisle leading to an altar. The walls were paneled wood and we were surprised that there were no crosses or religious iconography hanging on them. There were a variety of musical instruments; drums, an electric piano, tambourines, and acoustic and electric guitars set up behind the altar. Reverend Elkins told me he was a disabled coal miner whose family has lived in his beloved rugged mountains for generations and that he was one of several thousand serpent handlers living throughout Appalachia. He introduced me to another church elder, Dewey Chafin. The latter looked to be in his seventies. He had piercing blue eyes and hands that looked like claws with knotted and swollen fingers. He had been bitten by snakes more than a hundred times. We laid our coats and bags on the rearmost pews. Victorine unpacked her camera and began photographing the church's interior and its strict doctrine, which was handwritten on posters, hung on the wood paneled walls:

Women are not allowed to wear: short sleeves, jewelry, or make-up (I Peter 3:3, Timothy 2:9)

No gossiping (James 1:26)

No tale bearing (Proverbs 18:8)

No lying (Colossians 3:9, Revelation 21:8)

No backbiting (Romans 1:30)

No bad language or by-words (Colossians 3:8)

No tobacco users (II Corinthians 7:1; I Corinthians 3:17)

Men not allowed to have long hair, mustache, or beard (I Corinthians 11:14)

Men not allowed to wear short sleeves

Women not allowed to cut hair (I Corinthians 11:15), to wear dresses above knees (Timothy 2:9)

Five cedar boxes with Plexiglas covers secured with locks sat on a raised platform in front of the altar. Pastor Chafin beckoned us closer. Approximately twenty snakes were crawling in their boxes hissing and rattling at us menacingly from behind their Plexiglas covering. I shuddered and promised myself not to get too close to those frightening creatures. Snakes have always terrified me but these looked particularly nasty.

"These are rattlesnakes," he said, pointing out some black, yellow, and olive colored snakes with diamond shaped blotches.

"And these are copperheads," he said, pointing to four big beige and tan vipers.

Their bodies were covered with dark brown to reddish hourglass-shaped cross bands and their triangularly shaped heads had the color of an old copper coin. Rattlesnakes possess a set of fangs with which they inject large quantities of hemotoxic venom that travels through the bloodstream destroying tissue, causing swelling, internal bleeding, and intense pain. Some species, such as the Mojave Rattlesnake, also possess a neurotoxic component in their venom that causes paralysis and other nervous symptoms.

As Pastor Chafin introduced us to the snakes, I noticed that worshippers were slowly making their way into the church and quietly taking their places in the pews. I wondered which ones were going to be our hosts tonight. The women wore their hair long, sometimes pinned in a bun, ankle-length dresses and absolutely no cosmetics while the men had short hair and long-sleeved shirts. One by one musicians took their place on the stage behind the altar and began tuning their instruments. Everyone greeted us very politely and no one asked us who we were or what we were doing there—no gossip, I thought. These people came exclusively to receive God's blessing. I took my seat in the rear, close to the children with my notebook in my lap and my tape recorder on the bench next to me while Victorine valiantly stood up close to the snake boxes. I counted thirty-four women, men and children in attendance. Reverend Elkins began his sermon . . .

"We thank the Lord for everybody who's gathered here today. If'n you decide to handle the serpents, remember, you handle them on your own. If'n you get bit, you get bit on your own. Anybody's under age eighteen, don't go into the boxes, 'cuz I tell ya, there's death in them boxes. You hear me children? . . . there's death in them boxes. Now, let's everybody pray at this time. Everybody just come forward when you're ready, put everything you got into it and we could have a good blessing and Lord willin' we'll all go home blessed tonight. Alright now, everybody just pray right in."

Suddenly, all the members of the Church dropped to their knees in prayer, their eyes shut tight with elbows resting on the pews. "Amen." Pastor Dewey called out after a few minutes and the entire congregation answered in chorus, "AMEN." Suddenly, the band launched into a Rock-a-Billy rhythm that which sounded like an old Elvis Presley or Jerry Lee Lewis song played at roadhouse dance halls. The sound of the pounding drums, twangy electric guitars, and out-of-tune piano filled the air. The congregants started swaying and clapping their hands along with the music.

"What do ya think about Jesus?" sang Reverend Elkins.

"Yeah, he's all right," sang back the congregation in unison.

"What do ya think about Jesus?"

"Yeah, he's all right."

They repeated it over and over as the music grew louder and louder, building in intensity with each call and response. One by one, parishioners rose from their pews, made their way to the altar and began dancing, but not like any dancing I had ever seen before. They truly looked possessed. One woman spun in circles with her arms outstretched while a man next to her ran in place while he pumped his head and arms up and down, shouting and singing. A few people climbed onto the altar, pulled shakers and tambourines from a basket onstage, and joined in with the band.

On an unseen cue the music stopped and Reverend Elkins stepped up to the podium. A dozen parishioners stood before him, spinning and bowing and rocking side to side.

"Praise God," he proclaimed.

"Praise God," they chanted back.

"Praise God because he's worthy of all the praise."

"Praise God."

"Praise God because he's worthy of all the glory."

"Praise God, praise God tonight and he shall anoint you. Praise God and his spirit shall enter you and protect you from harm. He shall anoint you and nothin' will harm you."

The drummer pounded out four quick beats on his bass drum and the band launched into another song, louder and more foot-stompingly raucous than the last. A woman shrieked and as she fell backwards towards the floor, nearby parishioners caught and held her as her entire body began to shake violently, as if an electric current was coursing through it. She was helped to her knees, began bowing and waving her arms then began to speak . . .

"Shig de rah dada, rack te bah da! Shand da ba dee kee ri kee ra shi ding! Baba de shig te bah da, shing da kee ri!" she called, then collapsed back onto the floor.

I looked over to Victorine who had been taking photos but was now frozen in place with her mouth open and her eyes as big as saucers staring at the woman. After a moment she looked back at me with an expression of utter disbelief then went back to taking photos. I learned later that what the woman was doing was called glossolalia or "speaking in tongues," channeling the Holy Spirit through her and speaking an unknown language. The music grew louder and faster and almost the entire congregation was gyrating on the floor when the unbelievable happened. In the middle of his dancing, an elder walked up to the altar, unclasped the lid on one of the snake boxes and pulled out a four-foot black timber rattler that was rattling threateningly. Seemingly spellbound by the reptile, he stared at it intensely as he held it high in the air and spun in circles, faster and faster. He began chanting, "Praise Jesus! Praise Jesus! Praise Jesus!" Dumbfounded, I watched as other worshippers joyfully removed more snakes from the boxes and waved them in the air while bobbing and weaving in front of the altar. I nervously watched Victorine getting dangerously close to the serpents in her never-ending quest for the perfect photos. She was trying to catch close ups of the snakes with congregants dancing fiercely in the background.

A woman wearing a green jersey and a long black skirt unclasped the lid of another box, pulled out a tangle of four or five snakes and placed them on the floor. She danced around and over them in her bare feet, nudging them with her toes. I distinctly saw what looked like terror in her eyes but her faith was evidently stronger. She began twirling around, repeating, "Thank you, Lord, thank you, Lord Jesus, thank you, Lord, thank you, Lord Jesus, thank you . . ." and went on spinning slowly with the snakes at her feet in an implausible death dance. She then bent down, scooped them up, and passed them on to another grey-haired woman who went on dancing while looking at her reptilian partners with a mix of terror and awe.

Another elder clutched a snake in each hand as he danced, stomping his feet to the music which was now building to a feverish pitch. Perspiration dripped from his face. Completely stunned, I watched the serpent's forked tongue flicking up and down near the face of the worshipper whose eyes were closed, seemingly in a trance. Reverend Dewey Chafin gathered six rattlesnakes together and held them aloft with one hand in what seemed an act of both defiance and victory.

One man held a snake's head close to his forehead in a gentle caress. Another tall lanky man wearing a four-foot long rattlesnake around his neck like a scarf, spun in circles to the music. Reverend Elkins passed his snakes to a woman next to him, jumped up on the podium, grabbed the microphone and began to sing.

"Talkin' about Jesus," he called.

"We gonna have a good time," the congregation responded in time to the driving beat.

"Talkin' about Jesus . . ."

"We gonna have a good time . . ."

"Talkin' about Jesus . . ."

"We gonna have a good time . . ."

"Talkin' about Jesus . . ."

"We gonna have a good time . . ."

They repeated the call and response over and over. It reached a frenetic pace. Parishioners collapsed and writhed on the floor speaking in tongues. Were the snakes inhibited by the loud frenetic music? I have no idea, but I know that the scene that unfolded before our eyes was simply beyond belief.

More was yet to come as Pastor Dewey walked up to altar, ominously repeating, "If they drink any deadly thing, it shall not hurt them, if they drink any deadly thing, it shall not hurt them, if they drink any deadly thing, it shall not hurt them . . .". He grabbed a bottle filled with clear yellowish liquid that was sitting on the altar and took a generous swig. I blinked. Could it be the bottle of strychnine we had heard about? I expected him to collapse immediately but he went on singing and dancing. He handed the bottle to Reverend Elkins, who took a swig and began spinning in slow circles, jerking his head from side to side, slowly at first, then faster and faster.

"Hasha rum reeshi, hasha rum baba, Hasha rum reeshi, hasha rum baba, Hasha rum reeshi, hasha rum baba . . ." he chanted as he spun faster and faster. He finally collapsed in a heap on the floor, lay there for a moment then sprang to his knees and howled, "Praise God, he is worthy of all the glory!"

The band stopped suddenly, then began playing a hymn, a slow hymn, and the children in the pews next to me began to sing . . .

"This little light of mine, I'm gonna let it shine . . ."

One by one the parishioners gathered up the serpents and placed them back in their boxes, took seats in the pews and joined the children singing.

"This little light of mine, I'm gonna let it shine . . ."

Parishioners who had collapsed and were sprawled onto the floor slowly got to their feet, returned to their pews, and joined the singing.

"This little light of mine, I'm gonna let it shine, let it shine, let it shine, let it shine."

As the congregation repeated a few more choruses of the calming hymn, they slowly composed themselves and returned to the sedate state they were in when I first saw them enter the church. Reverend Elkins addressed the congregation from the altar.

"The spirit of the Lord has certainly touched us tonight. Take that spirit home with you and keep it in your hearts, goodnight."

I looked at my watch. Was it really ten p.m.? The service had lasted approximately three nerve-wracking hours. The parishioners smiled and nodded to me with serene glows on their faces as they quietly left the church. I was sitting there dazed, trying to understand the strange bliss these people seemed to experience flirting with their own death when Reverend Elkins, who was speaking to a benevolent-looking couple, caught my eye and motioned me towards him. I grabbed my notebook and recorder and joined him near the door. Victorine was still busy photographing at the altar in front of the church.

"Thank you for joinin' us tonight," said Reverend Elkins, "I hope you got all the information you need for your newspaper article."

"Yes, thank you," I answered, still trying to process in my mind all I had just witnessed.

"This is Brother John and his wife Eli," he said, introducing me to the couple next to him, "they are goin' to accommodate you tonight."

"It's a pleasure to meet you," I said shaking their hands, "My name is Natasha and that's my sister Victorine taking photographs."

I almost fainted when I saw that Eli was carrying one of the boxes of snakes and I realized our hostess was one of the women who had been handling them during the service. I wasn't too sure I liked the idea of being so close to these serpents. I thanked them for their kindness, complimented her on her courage, and asked them a few questions. As I spoke with them I noticed from the corner of my eye a tall lanky man who I remembered during the service had been wearing a rattlesnake around his neck like a scarf while spinning round and round. Now he was speaking softly to Reverend Elkins and repeatedly glancing up towards the altar where Victorine was finishing up taking photos. She packed up her camera and I watched him follow her intently with his eyes as she walked over to meet us.

"This is Brother John and his wife Eli," I said, "we'll be staying with them tonight."

"It's a pleasure to meet you," she said with a big smile, her eyes beaming, "I took some nice photos of you and your serpents when . . ."

The tall lanky man cleared his throat.

"Oh, yes . . . and this is Brother Abner," said Reverend Elkins.

Brother Abner stepped forward slightly. He stood fumbling with his hat in his hands, staring at the floor directly in front of Victorine.

"I noticed you taking photographs," he said.

Victorine looked at me then back to Abner.

"Yes, that right," she answered.

Abner glanced up at her face then quickly went back to staring at the floor as he continued to fumble with his hat.

"Do you like taking photographs?" he asked.

"Yes, most of the time. It depends on what I'm photographing," she answered.

"That's good," he answered still staring at the floor.

Brother John interrupted the uncomfortable silence that followed.

"Well, I guess we had better be gettin' on home," he said. "You ladies must be tired after your long drive from New York City."

"Yes, thank you John. I am a bit tired," I said, "Goodbye and thank you Reverend . . . and nice to meet you too Abner."

"Yes, thank you, goodbye," said Victorine as she turned and hurried to the door.

John and Eli loaded their snakes into the back of their pickup truck and as we pulled out of the parking lot to follow them to their home I turned to see Reverend Elkins and Brother Abner standing at the front door, watching us drive away.

"It looks like you have an admirer," I said.

"Be quiet. That's enough from you," she hissed.

"Did you see? It was so cute. He was smitten. He could barely speak, or even look at you," I said laughing.

"Well, it's too bad for him because he got his last look tonight. We'll be gone tomorrow, now be quiet, I'm trying to concentrate," she said, peering through the windshield, following the taillights ahead of us.

We arrived at John and Eli's home, which turned out to be a long rickety trailer parked on bare earth a few miles down the road from the church. As we entered I noticed duct tape–covered holes in the broken windows behind the faded curtains and worn linoleum covered the floor. On the couch lay a pillow with a picture of Niagara Falls and above it hung a reproduction of Leonardo da Vinci's *Last Supper* painted on velvet. It was already well past 10 p.m. and Eli quickly showed us to our bedroom, which we realized was actually theirs. We vainly protested but they wouldn't hear about letting us sleep on the sofa. Our hosts were actually some of the most caring people I have ever met. They even wanted to know what we wanted for breakfast.

"Oh, whatever you're having. We have been eating at highway rest stops so whatever you serve will feel like a five star hotel's breakfast to us," I answered with a smile.

We were lucky to be staying with these incredibly kind people. The nearest hotel was over one hour away from the church and I had no desire to take a chance driving at night on those serpentine dark mountain roads. The small bedroom in the rear of the trailer, just past the cramped bathroom, was just large enough to fit the bed, a closet, and a few cardboard boxes of books and clothes. It was obvious from the trailer's poor condition and its old worn interior that John and Eli were very poor. How touching though, we thought, that they were inviting us to stay at their more than modest home. Victorine drifted off to sleep quickly and was soon snoring softly next to me but I can't say that I slept very soundly. I awoke several times, terrified with an ominous feeling, unable to shake the vision of rattlesnakes and copperheads from my mind. I finally drifted off to sleep somewhere after 3 a.m. but was jolted awake at 7:30 a.m. by a knock on our bedroom door.

"Yes, come in," I answered. I looked over groggily at Victorine who was still fast asleep.

Eli tiptoed in, smiling. Her long blonde hair was up in a bun and she was wearing a blue flowered skirt and a grey blouse. She looked over and saw that Victorine was still asleep.

"Did you sleep well?" she whispered.

"Oh, very well, thank you so much," I lied.

"The snakes didn't bother you, I hope?" Eli said as she crouched down next our bed and began pulling something out from underneath it.

"No, not at all," I replied, my mind still clouded with sleep, not knowing what she meant exactly. Was she reading my dreams? I looked down at what she was doing and in one horrific flash I realized what she had meant. Eli had retrieved two of those same boxes she had carried to the church yesterday. The snakes were under our bed the entire night. I jumped backwards in the bed, on top of Victorine.

"*What are you doing? Get off of me,*" she cried.

"I'm glad they were quiet. Now I've got to feed them. I'll see you in the dining room. Breakfast will be ready in about thirty minutes," said Eli as she carried the boxes outside and pulled the door shut.

"*They were under our bed!*" I cried. "*The snakes were under our bed the entire night.*"

"*Did they bite you?*" she asked.

"*No,*" I answered shaking.

"*Then what's your problem? There's a first time for everything,*" she said, laughing at my horrified expression.

"*And the last time for me,*" I moaned, collapsing onto my pillow. I was still tired and yearned to be back in my own bed in New York City.

Half an hour later the smell of breakfast cooking filled the small trailer and we found John sitting at the table when we emerged from the bedroom. Eli was setting our plates on the table. It was a huge breakfast:

eggs, toast, and to Victorine's delight, grits. A large jar of grape jelly also sat on the table next to another filled with instant coffee, which John was stirring into his mug.

"Grits! Yum, I love grits," said Victorine, who sat down and began eating immediately.

"Would you like some scrapple?" asked Eli.

"Scrapple?" asked Victorine. "What's scrapple?"

"Pork scraps mixed with corn meal," answered Eli. "It's made from what's left over after we butcher a pig."

"Everything but the oink," added John.

Eli placed a helping of scrapple on Victorine's plate but I declined. Victorine took a bite and immediately smiled.

"It tastes like grandmaman's andouillettes," said Victorine.

Although the food smelled delicious I couldn't find my appetite. I was trying to be nonchalant as I scanned the room, looking for those two terrifying boxes. Eli must have noticed my anxiety and read my mind.

"Don't worry dear. The serpents are outside in the sun where they can stay warm," she reassured me.

"Oh, thank you," I said, letting out a sigh of relief.

With the snakes safely outside I relaxed and began to eat my breakfast. It was a huge plate of food I didn't think I could finish. Victorine on the other hand was practically inhaling her food and everything on her plate was almost gone.

"Oh careful, I think you missed a piece of scrapple," I teased.

She glared at me, obviously offended.

"How many kilos have you gained since we got to America?"

"I don't know. You eat a lot too," she snapped back defensively with her mouth full. It was true, I'm ashamed to admit, but America had changed our eating habits. Worse than that, it had changed our relationship to food. We were now eating mindlessly, but I was tired and a bit cranky from lack of sleep. I couldn't resist teasing her some more.

"You're beginning to look like the Michelin Man's wife."

Victorine ignored me. I could tell I had upset her. She turned to Eli with a forced smile.

"So, when did you start snake handling?" she asked.

"Oh, I had pious God-fearing parents who passed it on to me. I've been around it my whole life. John's story is a little different," Eli replied, turning to him.

"For me it came much later. I'm a Marine veteran. After I got out of the service I found I was becoming mean and drinkin' a lot. I hit bottom, rock bottom and was afraid of goin' to hell. Then one day I met Eli and she helped bring the spirit of God in my life. It changed me completely."

We learned that like most of Jolo's male inhabitants, John was a retired coal miner who, like Reverend Elkins, had worked in the coal mines for thirty years and consequently spent a good part of his life in the dark.

"Were you scared when first handled the snakes?" I asked him.

"I'd lie if I said I weren't scared. I hate snakes. They're evil," said John.

"But, when you're anointed and filled with the spirit of the Lord, there's nothin' that can hurt you," said Eli, "I've never been bit but John has, once on his hand. Show them, John."

John held out his hand and showed us the scarred tissue.

"What happened?" I asked.

"He was takin' a serpent from the box but the spirit of the Lord wasn't truly in him, he wasn't protected, the serpent knew it and struck him. His whole arm swolled up, he lost a lot of blood and he had problems breathin'. It took a whole year to heal," she explained.

She rummaged in her cupboard and pulled out an envelope filled with photos.

"This first picture was taken about an hour after the strike," said Eli. "The blood under the skin immediately started to boil, causing blood blisters to form on the hand."

In the second photo we were able to see blood blisters forming high up his arm.

"The blisters were swellin' up real quick due to the venom moving up the bloodstream," explained Eli, "and those blisters were popping and throwing blood around the room. By this time his arm had swolled up like a balloon."

"In this last picture here you can see that the skin on over half of John's arm is gone, completely gone," said Eli, "and the scar tissue is the same as that from a third-degree burn."

"I have full use of my hand now though and it is about almost as strong as it was before," said John, opening and closing his fist, "that was a year and half ago."

"The pain must have been terrible," I said.

"Oh, the pain was somethin' awful but sometimes the Lord lets the snake bite to remind us that the danger's real," John explained.

Just then I heard a vehicle outside. It sounded like it was pulling into the driveway. It made an awful racket, like it had a hole in its muffler.

"That sounds like Abner's truck," said Eli, cocking her head to the side.

Victorine's eyes got bigger as she sat up straight. John pulled back the curtain and looked out the window.

"Yup, that's Abner's truck alright," he said, "I wonder what he wants?"

"Yes, I wonder what he wants." I said turning to Victorine with a mischievous smile.

We heard the engine stop, the truck door open and shut, then footsteps approaching the trailer. They stopped just outside the door. There was a long pause. John, Eli and I looked at each other quizzically. I looked at Victorine sitting bolt upright. Her eyes were closed and she had a pained look on her face. Finally, there was a knock on the trailer door and Eli reached over to open it. Outside stood Abner, with his hair neatly combed and a large manila envelope in his hand.

"Good mornin', Abner. Would you like to come in?" asked Eli.

"I'd be much obliged, thank you," said Abner.

He stepped inside the already crowded trailer and closed the door behind him.

"Good morning Abner," said John, "how can we help you?"

"I hope I'm not disturbin' you," he replied.

"No, not at all," said Eli, "we just finished breakfast and were talkin' to Natasha and Victorine. We were just showing them the pictures you took of John's hand."

"That's good," said Abner, looking down at his manila envelope.

"Pictures you took? Abner, are you a photographer?" I asked.

Abner's ears and cheeks flushed bright red as he nodded his head.

"Well then, you and Victorine have something in common," I said, turning to Victorine with grin. I caught her eye and could tell from her look that she was in no mood for me to have any more fun at her expense. She jumped in and took control of the conversation.

"Oh really? What kind of camera do you use Abner?" she asked, offering her sweetest smile.

"An Argus C3," he replied, staring at her coffee mug.

"Wow, really?" she asked, sounding sincerely surprised, "how long have you had it?"

"As long as I can remember," he answered. "It's my father's camera. He gave it to me before he passed." He slowly looked up into Victorine's eyes. "It's in the truck. Would you like to see it?" he asked.

"Yes, I would," she said, "let me grab my camera and we'll come outside. How does that sound?"

"That's good," he answered, nodding quickly.

We pulled on our jackets, Victorine grabbed her camera bag, and we followed Abner outside as Eli cleared the breakfast dishes. Abner opened the passenger door on his rusted pickup truck. Sitting on the seat was a bundle wrapped in a plaid blanket. He opened it and inside was a rectangular leather carrying case. He removed it from the truck, opened it, carefully removed an ancient-looking black camera and handed it to Victorine. She examined it carefully as Abner watched.

"Abner, this is a fine camera. You've obviously taken very good care of it," said Victorine carefully handing it back to him, "You still use it?"

"Yes," said Abner, "My father taught me how to clean and maintain it. It still works and he always said, 'If it ain't broke, don't fix it.' My father taught me everything about photography."

Abner tucked his camera back into its case and placed it back in the truck. He picked up the manila envelope he was holding when he arrived and turned to Victorine.

"If it's not too much trouble, I mean, if you don't mind, I would like to see some of the photographs you took at the church last night. I wrote my address on this envelope here and I put some extra stamps on it too. Maybe you could send me some prints that you like."

He held the manila envelope out to her and a gentle smile came to his face as she took it from him.

"Of course Abner, I'd be happy to," she said. "Few people go to this much trouble of giving me an envelope already addressed and stamped. It would be my pleasure."

Abner's face lit up as his ears and cheeks flushed red again.

"Thank you, thank you kindly," he said.

"So Abner, how long have you been a photographer?" I asked.

"Oh, I've been takin' pictures ever since I was little," he answered, "My father bought me a Brownie camera when I was ten years old. I still have that camera too. My father taught me everything about photography."

Abner seemed kind and gentle-natured like the other parishioners we had met. I decided to ask him a few questions for our article.

"Are you originally from Jolo?" I asked.

"No, I grew up down the road in Coalwood," he answered. "We lost the house after my father passed. That's when my mother and I moved here. I take care of her now."

"How long ago was that?" I asked.

"Fifteen years," he said.

"When did you start attending the Church of Lord Jesus?" I asked.

"I met Reverend Elkins at the store right after we moved in," he said, "He invited me to attend service at his church."

"Was that the first time you had been to a church where people handled serpents?" I asked.

"Yes, we were Baptist back in Coalwood. The first time, I'll tell you, it was the strangest thing I ever saw and I got scared. I didn't go back right away but somethin' kept pulled at me. I couldn't stay away. I know now it was the spirit of the Lord pullin' me."

"You felt pulled back?" I asked.

"Yes, when I went back the second time, I knew I was truly touched by the spirit of the Lord," he answered as his eyes grew wider. "It's hard to explain but when that spirit of the Lord touches you, there's no better feelin' in the world. It's like a bucket of cool water hittin' you on a hot summer day. Colors look different, everything disappears around you and you feel like you are in another world. "

"Does your mother attend church with you?" I asked.

The light suddenly left Abner's face. He looked down at his feet and shook his head.

"No," he answered, "My mother won't go to church no more, not since my father passed. She don't talk no more and don't want to get out of bed into her wheelchair no more either."

My breakfast suddenly felt like a stone in my stomach. Victorine and I exchanged glances.

"Is it just you and your mother?" asked Victorine.

"That's right," he answered softly.

"It must be difficult without any help," I said.

"No, I promised my father I'd take care of her," he said standing up a bit straighter, "The strength of the Lord's all the help I need."

"Of course, of course, I understand," I said.

Victorine thankfully jumped in and quickly changed the subject back to photography.

"What sorts of things do you like to photograph, Abner?"

Abner looked down at his feet then back up to Victorine.

"I like to photograph things that people don't see," he said looking straight into her eyes. "A lot of people don't notice things right in front of them."

Victorine crossed her arms, leaned against the fender of our car, took a long look at Abner and nodded her head.

"I'd like to see some more of your photographs," she said, "besides those of John's hand."

"Would you really?" he asked.

"Yes, really," she said, nodding with a gentle smile.

"Well, I meant it to be a surprise for you to find when you got home, but, well, that envelope I gave you there, it's not empty, I put three of my photographs inside," he said as his ears and cheeks blushed even redder than before.

"Really? In this envelope?" she said holding up the large manila envelope he had given her.

Abner nodded. Victorine opened the flap on the envelope, looked inside, pulled out the photographs, and looked at them one by one as Abner watched her intently. Her eyes grew wide. She looked up at him then back to the photographs and I could tell that she was truly surprised.

"*Natasha, come look at these,*" she said to me, then to Abner, "Abner, these are beautiful. I can tell you do see what a lot of people miss."

She handed me the photographs: three eight by ten-inch, black and white prints. It was true. The photos were beautiful. The first: a close up of two coal miners side by side, surrounded by darkness, their upturned faces blackened with soot, squinting into beams of sunlight shining from above. The second: a hunched old woman in a tattered winter coat, walking away from the camera pulling a large basket of groceries down a long dirt road, no house or perceivable destination in site. The third: a landscape, a deep valley, steep tree-covered hills rising sharply on either side. The bottom of the valley filled like a tub with a thick layer of fog and the early morning sun bathing its smooth surface with an otherworldly silvery glow. Out of the fog poked a church steeple and a water tower, both casting long shadows on its surface.

"Abner," I exclaimed, "these are wonderful."

"Yes, just beautiful . . . Where do you do your processing?" asked Victorine.

"You mean develop my film?" he asked, looking puzzled.

"Yes, and your prints," she added.

"My dark room is in the basement," he said.

"You do all your film and print processing yourself?" she asked, her eyes wide.

"Yes, my father taught me everything about photography," he answered.

"He certainly did, Abner, he certainly did, but it's your eye that sees those images and captures them," she said, "no one can teach you that."

He looked down at the ground and shifted uneasily on his feet.

"I guess you're right about that," he said, "I'm glad you like them."

"Thank you, it's the nicest gift I've received in a long time," she said. "When I send you the photos I took last night, I'm going to include some other photos of mine . . ."

He looked up. A huge smile covered his entire face.

" . . . and I'm going to send a self-addressed envelope of my own. I'm hoping that you'll write back to me and tell me what you think . . ."

Abner nodded.

" . . . and you have to promise to be honest, okay?"

"Oh, I will," he said.

"Good, now what do you say we take a few photographs," said Victorine. "Let's use my camera."

We spent a few minutes taking turns photographing each other in front of his pickup, then Abner said he had to get back to check on his mother. We waved goodbye to him as his truck sputtered out of the driveway. Once he was out of sight we went back inside the trailer to say thank you and goodbye to our hosts, John and Eli.

"We want to thank you for opening your home to us. We'd like to give you something for your trouble," I said.

"Oh, no," said John, "no trouble at all."

"It's only right to give shelter to a traveler in need," said Eli.

Just the same, when we went to pick up our bags in the bedroom, we made the bed and tucked a thank you note with forty dollars under the pillow. We were on the road by eleven a.m. and drove in silence as we wound back through the mountains down route sixteen towards the interstate. I was deep in thought. I felt I had a better sense of that bizarre religious practice and its symbolic meaning. It was obvious that to them, snake handling was a rite of passage that brought them closer to God and to holiness. As Eli had told us, snakes represent evil and Satan. Therefore, by exposing themselves to danger they were enacting the literal word of God, as a demonstration of their faith. Still, another aspect of the service intrigued me.

"*You know,*" I said, breaking our silence, turning to Victorine, "*if you take away the snakes and the strychnine, that church service was still pretty wild.*"

"*Yeah?*" said Victorine, "*and?*"

"*Well, think about it,*" I said, "*just imagine going to a place a few times a week, where you can sing and shout at the top of your lungs, dance and spin around on the floor like a banshee then jump up and start babbling nonsense words.*"

"*Yeah?*" said Victorine again, "*and?*"

"*Well, all your neighbors are doing the same thing,*" I said, "*no one is judging you. You can act crazy. Let go of stress. Maybe release a few demons . . . it would be good for you.*"

"*What? Good for me?*" asked Victorine laughing, "*Good for me to get rid of my demons? And you have none of your own?*"

We both laughed and practiced speaking in tongues as we drove down the winding mountain roads.

Cornmeal scrapple
Serves 6

- 1 cup of cornmeal, white or yellow
- 1 cup of milk
- 1 teaspoon of brown sugar
- 1 teaspoon of salt
- 2 cups of water
- 8 ounces bulk pork sausage, cooked and crumbled
- 2 tablespoons of butter
- 2 tablespoons of flour

1. Combine the cornmeal, milk, sugar, and salt. Stir occasionally and cook until thick. Cover and lower heat for 10 more minutes. Stir in the pork and remove from the heat.
2. Pour into greased mold, cover and refrigerate for 1 hour.
3. Remove it from its mold and cut into ⅓ in slices. Dip both slices in flour.
4. Melt butter in a pan and brown scrapple on both sides.

Moules Frites
Serves 4

- 4 pounds live mussels
- ¾ cup white wine (any kind of white)
- 1 tablespoon unsalted butter
- 1 chopped shallot
- 2 cloves chopped garlic

1. Scrub the mussels before cooking them. Only keep the closed mussels and set aside the ones that are open. If they close after a short time, then add them to the rest.
2. Heat the butter over medium-high heat in a large pot.
3. Sauté the shallot until it is soft but not browned and add the garlic cloves.
4. Add the white wine and bring it to a simmer.
5. Add the mussels. Cover the pot and let the mussels steam for 3–8 minutes.
6. After three minutes, check the mussels; many should be open, you want all of them open.
7. Cover for a minute and spoon them in individual bowls with plenty of broth.
8. Throw out any mussels that did not open.
9. Serve with homemade French fries.

Chapter Eight

In Dog We Trust

O ur next reportage was even more atypical than the previous ones. After doing a story on the transformation of the Ku Klux Klan, which, according to the Southern Poverty Law Center's director Mark Potok, had started to associate with pro-fascist groups, I discovered that the famously radical American feminist movement had somehow also affected the least likely to be affected, the KKK women. The KKK women did much more than just sew their husbands' robes ever since David Duke opened the doors of the movement to them. A former Imperial Wizard of Lousiana, Duke won 60 percent of the white votes when he ran for governor of Louisiana in 1992. Now armed, trained, and sometimes dressed in "battledress," KKK women had caught up with men and were actively taking part in the movement despite its pro-claimed hatred of feminism.

In 2000, the year of our magazine article, women accounted for forty percent of the Klan's membership compared to only twenty-five percent in other neo-Nazi organizations. According to New York's Grand Dragon, James Sheeley, this development was purely pragmatic: men had understood they needed women to insure the KKK's survival. Still, we had a perfect angle for a story: the KKK women's increased role in the movement. The modern Invisible Empire, a.k.a. the KKK, a far right organization which advocated white supremacy, white nationalism, anti-immigration, had splintered into 179 chapters and the largest and most active one was the American Knights of Ku Klux Klan in Indiana. The magazine's editor was very enthusiastic and, after receiving her blessing and some much-needed money to cover our expenses, we got the project started.

The pressures were very intense since it was our first big reportage for *Marie France,* a respected, high-profile magazine. We were understandably on edge. However, the approach was easier than we thought. Cecile, another French reporter and good friend of mine from university had done a story on the KKK in Ohio, where Ohio's Grand Dragon, Reverend Hogg, had admitted her to the KKK Convention and, after having duly searched her and her car, let her ask his members questions. Reverend Hogg was apparently in close contact with Indiana's Imperial Wizard (Klan jargon for "overall leader"), Jeffrey Berry. Cecile had vouched for us and after numerous correspondence between Reverend Hogg, Jeffrey Berry, and myself, he was reassured that we were trustworthy. Did Hogg also tell him that we were two young naïve and harmless French reporters? It is possible. In any case, we received the most improbable invitation, one that would have probably delighted many American reporters, one that no reporter could ever refuse: an invitation to spend a weekend on Reverend Berry's property in Newsville, Indiana, with the American Knights of the Ku Klux Klan.

Were we crazy? Not quite. Did we fear for our lives? Perhaps a little bit. Did we have an emergency plan in case something happened? Not yet. How would they react in front of two French women who lived in New York City? Would our presence make them feel somehow suspicious? In truth, we weren't too sure ourselves but we knew we had to work on reassuring them tacitly to get some good insights into their lives. So, during the eleven-hour highway drive, we "rehearsed" intensely on how to approach the dreaded KKK women.

"*We can always tell them that we are members of Le Pen's Front National,*" Victorine shrewdly suggested.

Le Pen's Front National was France's far right political party with an ideology some might say teetered perilously close to the KKK's.

"You do the talking. I'll keep quiet," I answered, mortified at the thought of being found out as left wing intruders in a far right enclave.

To me, Le Pen was off limits but I guess Victorine didn't have my political scruples. Or maybe she was a partisan of "the end justifies the means."

"I'll tell the campground's manager to call the police if they don't see us come back in the evening," she said portentously. I gave her an anxious look. She seemed serious. She was starting to make me really nervous so I remained quiet to prevent her from fueling my increasing anxiety but Victorine apparently had some old scores to settle with me.

"We must try not to raise any suspicions so for once in your life, try not to act like a princess. Don't refuse to eat the food they offer you. Remember we're invited to their picnic. A picnic is an occasion where people eat," she warned me sarcastically.

"What do you mean a 'princess'? I never behaved like a princess in my life!" I snapped back. She had hurt my feelings and was now relentless.

"Oh come on. You've always acted like you are better than anybody else. Even when we were little you always got away with not doing the dishes pretending you had to study for a test. I always ended up doing the dishes while you'd go read in your bedroom," she snapped.

"What!?"

"Oh please, don't act dumb. Maman always let you get away with it just because you got better grades. You got away with everything," she said lowering the radio, preparing for an argument.

I had no idea where all this was coming from. Victorine was in the mood to fight and I was starting to lose my temper.

"Well, if I was the princess, you were the queen. When I think about all that money Papa spent buying you Figaro . . ."

"WHAT! . . . Yes, Figaro was my stallion but Papa was also riding him. Besides, how was I supposed to lead riding classes without a horse? I was working, WORKING for the family business . . . and it's not my fault if you were too scared to put your ninny behind on him," she hissed.

"Keep your eyes on the road, you're going to get us in an accident," I screamed as the car started to drift over the yellow line.

I couldn't believe it. Frankly, she had chosen the worse time for a confrontation, just before our scheduled weekend with the KKK, when I had butterflies in my stomach. I decided to ignore her cantankerous attacks and looked out the window as she continued.

"It was always that way. Whenever any work had to be done, you would disappear into you room . . . and your excuse? . . . 'I have to study, I have to study'," she continued in a mocking tone, *"And Maman and Papa always fell for it . . ."*

I was getting very upset by now and had to hold my tongue. I was about to get very nasty and almost said that if this was the bitchy way she acted with Nigel, her now ex-boyfriend, it was no wonder he cheated on her, but I held back. The details of that subject had been off limits since she returned from London; a closed door she refused to open, even to our mother to whom we usually told everything. I knew it was an open wound and no matter how upset I was or how much she was provoking me, it was best not to pour salt on it. I breathed deeply, tuned her out, and continued staring out the window as she muttered to herself. Finally she relented and increased the volume of the radio.

When we reached a rest stop in Ohio, we hadn't spoken for almost three hours but my anger had receded and I could tell that Victorine's had also. We bought burgers and chips and sat silently eating them while sitting at one of the outdoor picnic tables. Suddenly Victorine froze and I noticed her staring over my shoulder with a horrified look on her face. She sprang up from her seat and ran out into the busy parking lot. I turned to see her running towards a black puppy that was darting between the passing cars obviously confused and terrified.

"Oh no, don't tell me you're lost," she said tenderly as the puppy crouched down, tail between his legs and gratefully let her pet him. Victorine had a way of making any animal she was near feel safe.

Dodging the traffic in the parking lot I ran to join Victorine and the puppy and started stroking him too. He looked to be about four months old, was entirely black with little pointed ears and amazingly humanlike eyes. I looked around. Nobody appeared to be looking for a stray dog.

I went inside the gas station to enquire about the puppy but nobody had made any request.

"I'll bet he's been abandoned. We get that here a lot," said the blonde blue-eyed girl behind the register.

"That's it. We have no choice. We have to take him with us and try to get him some nice owners," Victorine said decisively. I nodded in agreement. Saving the dog's life was an emergency and our animosity towards each other had vanished. He gobbled up what remained of our burgers and then, since he wasn't very clean, we used our towels to fashion a little bed for him on the backseat. Gazing up at us with his big expressive eyes, the puppy looked adorable. Once we were back on the road he was soon fast asleep.

As usual, Victorine had dealt with the logistics. She had chosen a beautiful Christian campground located twenty miles from our meeting place in pastoral Indiana. The campground was huge with tall pine and sycamore trees and of course a few crosses. Nobody was there to tell us where to set up our tent so we chose the perfect spot near a wooden picnic table and benches among majestic sycamore trees. After we set up camp Victorine went to the bathroom to wash the pup while I sat at the table breathing the pure air and enjoying the serene environment. I noticed a breeze was starting to pick up and dark clouds gathering in the sky. Victorine returned carrying the puppy accompanied by a bubbly elderly lady dressed in a T-shirt, shorts, and leather sandals.

"Natasha, this is Betty Jo, whom I just had the pleasure of meeting in the bathroom. I told her the puppy's story and she wants to help us. She's also offered to watch the puppy while we do our interview."

"Hello Natasha, nice to meet you. You have chosen the perfect campground. My husband and I have come here every year for the last ten years. We are retired, you see, born again Christians. The good Lord has blessed us with that privilege," she said, raising her eyes to the sky.

"It is a very nice campground," I said, wondering why Victorine had an odd smile on her face. I was soon to learn that born again Christians were a very different species from the snake handlers.

"We volunteer to take care of the grounds and make sure that this place remains a loving environment for the children of God."

Victorine had evidently found some very loving people, whom she was hoping would provide the puppy a new home.

"We're very happy to spend a couple of nights here and it would be wonderful if we could find some loving people for the blessed stray puppy we just found," I heard myself say, surprised at my own words.

"Dear Lord, Victorine told me about this lovely dog. How can people be so cruel? They really need to ask for help of God to repair their dark souls. Let's pray for that lovely loving dog," she said, joining her hands and closing her eyes for a few seconds. I looked at Victorine, wondering what to do but she remained stoical waiting for Betty Jo to finish and open her eyes.

"My very good friend just lost a small dog in a terrible way, bless the poor dog's soul. You might have been sent by God to replace her poor loving puppy. I will see what I can do to help you and your poor loving puppy," she said before departing.

We held our breath till she was gone then burst out laughing when she was out of sight. Were our own prayers going to be answered though Betty Jo? We looked at the puppy, full of hope.

A light rain began to fall as we were finishing our dinner. By the time we got into our tent, zipped up our flap, and were tucked into our sleeping bags with the puppy between us, it was pouring down hard. Soon the wind picked up and there was a constant barrage of thunder and lightning. I lay awake for hours, terrified by the storm. Lovie, as we had now started calling him, kept whining and fretting, making it very clear that he wanted to get out.

"*Maybe he wants to pee,*" said Victorine, nestled in her sleeping bag, making no move to take him out. Finally, around two a.m., I summoned up my courage and muttering under my breath, got up, unzipped the tent flap and went out with the flashlight into the torrential rain. Immediately Lovie ran away from me, I followed him, cursing, soaking wet. He hadn't peed or pooed. He was just sitting next to the car looking at it, indicating to me he wanted to get in.

"*OK, I know what you want . . .*" I said looking at the dripping tent, which seemed about to fly away.

"*You might have a point,*" I said scooping up Lovie and carrying him to the tent.

"Lovie wants to sleep in the car and frankly, I think I'd it prefer too," I called to Victorine.

I gathered my things, ran back to the car with Victorine close behind and once settled inside, totally exhausted, we finally fell asleep around five a.m.

The next thing I knew I was awakened abruptly by Lovie's barking and frantic knocking on the car's window.

"THANK YOU LORD! THANK YOU LORD!" I heard a muffled voice screaming.

I peered through the window and saw it was Betty Jo. Tears were streaming down her face as she cried, "Thank you for that miracle Lord. You saved those two loving girls by directing them to sleep in their car. Thank you for the miracle. Glory to the Lord!"

"What is it? What's going on now?" Victorine moaned peevishly.

Wiping the sleep from my eyes I stepped out of the car into the sunshine. The rain had stopped but the muddy ground was soaked with puddles, small fallen branches and leaves scattered everywhere. I looked past Betty Jo to our campsite. A few tree branches had fallen around us and I stared in disbelief at an enormous tree limb, slashed by lightning, lying across the middle of our flattened tent.

"I don't believe it," I said dumbfounded while Victorine stood frozen with her eyes wide and mouth hanging open.

Victorine turned to me slowly and in a quavering voice said, *"I think . . . I think Lovie saved our lives."*

We both stood watching Lovie who was now running in circles around our smashed tent barking and growling. He tentatively sniffed at it then came running back and sat down between us. Victorine picked him up, buried her nose in the fur behind his ears and cooed softly. Betty Jo stood next to us and repeatedly thanked the Lord for the miracle she believed he had accomplished, then scurried over to the little group of people who had begun gathering around to gawk at our tent. She grabbed the hand of one of the older gentlemen and led him back to where we were standing.

"This is Bob, my loving husband of forty-five blessed years, thank the Lord."

"Nice to meet you, Bob," we both said, still a bit stunned.

"Hello, I'm very happy to meet two lovely girls like yourselves. You certainly are two blessed loving creatures that Jesus put on our path to accomplish more good in this world. Betty Jo told me the whole story about the abandoned pup and how the Lord stepped in to repair the damage, just like he accomplished this miracle today. We won't condemn those who did this ugly thing and can only hope that Christ will teach them how to love again because Christ loves those that are unlovable. He knows how to walk with someone that betrays him and still can love them regardless, thank You Jesus for being our mighty Lord, both the Lion and the Lamb."

Bob was even more voluble than Betty Jo. Maybe I was a bit giddy from our near-death experience but I found myself about to laugh any second, so I precipitously reached into my pocket for a tissue and pretended to sneeze. I knew I couldn't look at Victorine. If I did my laughter would be irrepressible.

"Well, thank you Bob," said Victorine, "All this is very true and the coincidence that brought us here . . ."

She was immediately interrupted by Bob.

"No, no, no, it wasn't a coincidence, Victorine. The Lord knew what he was doing. I don't know if you truly understand the heart and mind of the God of Abraham, Isaac, and Jacob. God is Love. I want to encourage you to seek Him out for yourself. He wrote us love letters I call the Bible. It's not about a religion; it's about a relationship. I want to share his word and his love with you so you will know and see that God is good."

"Yes," Victorine answered coldly.

I sensed she was losing her patience and realized it was time to conclude our meeting for fear of jeopardizing our new relationship and losing a chance to find a home for Lovie.

"Victorine here is about to faint if she doesn't have breakfast after our ordeal. We have an important interview this afternoon, so maybe we shouldn't dally," I said, hoping, praying they didn't invite us to breakfast. Indeed, as lovely as they were, it was a torture to have to suppress my laughter. Even the snake handlers didn't speak like them. We had to remember to ask them which church they belonged to. We gave Lovie to Betty Jo and thanked them profusely.

"We will see you when we come back," I said.

"God willing, we will see you later, girls. I will talk to my friend about Lovie," Betty Jo promised.

Once in the car we burst into irrepressible laughter. Each time we look at each other or started to speak a new fit of giddiness overtook us. Once Victorine composed herself enough to drive we left to find a store to buy a new tent for the night.

Macaroni and Cheese
Serves 4

- 1 packet of macaroni (preferably organic)
- 4 tablespoons butter, melted
- 1 small onion, finely chopped
- 1 teaspoon salt
- ⅛ teaspoon ground black pepper
- 1½ cups milk
- 8 ounces (2 cups) Cheddar cheese, shredded

1. Boil water in a saucepan, and then add the macaroni. Once it is cooked drain well.
2. Preheat oven to 350°F. Grease 9-inch square baking or casserole dish. Set aside.
3. Add 4 tablespoons of butter over medium heat.
4. Add onion and cook until soft, about 5 minutes.
5. Add salt and pepper; stir until blended.
6. Stir in milk; cook, stirring, until thickened.
7. Remove from heat; stir in cheese.
8. Spoon macaroni into prepared baking dish.
9. Pour cheese sauce over macaroni.
10. Bake until bubbly and top is golden, about 20 minutes.
11. Let stand 15 minutes for easier serving.

Belgium endives with a Béchamel sauce
(Endives au jambon et à la sauce Béchamel)

- 8 Belgian endives
- 8 thin slices baked ham
- 8 ounces of Swiss cheese, grated
- 6 tablespoons of butter
- 3 tablespoons of flour
- 4 cups of milk
- A pinch of grated nutmeg
- Salt and pepper

1. Wash the endives and cut off the base.
2. Cook the endives in a steamer for about 8 minutes, drain them well, and cut the small, stubby ends.
3. Roll each endive in a slice of ham and place them in a buttered baking dish.
4. Pour the entire Béchamel sauce on top of the endives and cover them with the grated Swiss cheese on top.
5. Place the dish in the oven at 350°F for 20 minutes.

Béchamel sauce:

1. Melt the butter in a sauce pan at medium heat.
2. Add the flour into the melted butter and stir well with a whisk until smooth.
3. Stir in the milk a little at a time briskly to avoid lumps.
4. Continue to whisk, adding more milk until the sauce becomes creamy.
5. Reduce the heat to low and let it simmer for a few minutes whisking it occasionally.
6. Add the salt, pepper, and the nutmeg.

Chapter Nine

Ladies of the Knights—The Shooting Gallery

It was exactly three p.m. when we parked among the myriad of cars and pickups which were already clustered around the entrance to Reverend Berry's compound. If we had to make a quick getaway our car would be easy to find because it was the only one without a Confederacy flag decal stuck to it. My heart was beating fast as we followed the gravel driveway to the entrance gate. There we introduced ourselves to a high-strung armed guard, a young man dressed all in black with KKK insignias, tattoos, and mirrored sunglasses. His duty was to search people before letting them through and he was taking it very seriously. After carefully searching our bags and frisking us for weapons, he called over another security guard, a large tattooed blonde woman wearing black combat boots, black pants, a gun in a holster attached to her belt, and a T-shirt with a badge that read

Knight Hawk Security. She removed her mirrored sunglasses and looked at us suspiciously before curtly ordering us to follow her. She wasn't very friendly.

Reverend Berry's compound was large. Confederate flags were flying everywhere. Off to our right in a big empty field were two longhaired, tattooed men with chainsaws. They were cutting a huge tree trunk and making an awful din. To our left approximately a hundred people were sitting chatting at umbrella topped picnic tables while others tended nearby barbecue grills and children ran around playing and screaming. Except for all the guns, it was a reassuring pastoral scene . . . one big KKK family. The strong sun coupled with my highly emotional state wasn't helping me focus so it took me a few minutes to notice that the two lumberjacks were constructing the cross that was going to be burned later that evening in true KKK spirit. A huge pile of firewood lay in the adjacent field not far from the picnickers. As we worriedly studied the area, a blond bearded giant of a man suddenly loomed up in front of us. I stepped backward in awe. The man wore a leather vest over his T-shirt, black denim jeans, combat boots, and a gun in a holster attached to his belt. If this was Reverend Berry, he was the least monastic-looking reverend I had ever met in my life.

"I'm Reverend Berry. I'm guessing you're the two reporters from France," he said in a not so friendly way, his piercing blue eyes examining us.

"Yes, this is Natasha and I am Victorine. Thank you very much for inviting us to the Indiana KKK convention, or should I say 'Konvlocation'?" Victorine said, trying to break the ice with humor. Poor Victorine, she had tried to make a joke using Klan jargon but to no avail. Reverend Berry wasn't impressed with her sense of humor.

"Before you start walking around my property and interviewing my people, let me tell you what the rules are: one of my security men will be keeping an eye on you at all times. You are not allowed to take photos of children, of women, or of armed members. You may only take photos of people when they are wearing the hood. They will be wearing them at the cross burning tonight. You are not allowed to ask people their names either. If you defy my orders, your films will be confiscated and you will be kicked off of the property. Do you understand what I said?" he asked in a baritone voice that gave me the chills.

"Yes, we certainly do," Victorine answered.

From the corner of my eye, I observed the "security man." It was the mean-looking woman. She seemed determined to stay close to us at all times. I sensed she was going to plague us the whole time. I was hoping Victorine's charm would bring down her strong defenses and enable me to interview her. Reverend Berry was staring at me and I was getting slightly uncomfortable.

"Can't you talk?" he asked looking directly at me.

"Well, yes, yes, of course . . ." I blurted out, flustered.

"Good. You're welcome to help yourselves to the food. You will be allowed to ask me some questions later on," Reverend Berry concluded in a somewhat grandiloquent manner, signaling us we were now free to go.

We hesitated for a moment then walked down to the picnic tables tailed by our "security man." We introduced ourselves to a group of women sitting at one of the picnic tables as others around studied us with impenetrable faces. While they ate I stood next to the table and asked my first question.

"It seems that women have become more and more actively involved in the Klan nowadays. I guess we can say that they have become more empowered during the last five years. This is something fascinating to our female readers. Most of them have never even held a gun in their hands," I said feeling instinctively that the gun issue would be a good way to start the conversation. Indeed, a few women stepped closer to us, apparently intrigued.

"You can't carry a gun in France?" a young woman asked, looking up from her plate, her mouth full of chicken. She seemed genuinely surprised.

"Only hunters are allowed to carry guns and even then it's highly regulated, which is a real shame. Obviously, one needs to defend oneself in a dangerous world like ours," Victorine replied while I sighed heavily in dismay.

One woman whistled in horror. Another one looked at us with an air of deep sympathy as she patted the picnic bench next to her, inviting us to sit down. We sat next to them and I took out my notebook from my pants pocket.

"So, how did your involvement with the Klan start?" I asked, looking around at the group of women.

A young woman with short red hair and thin metal-rimmed glasses looked around at the other guests, then back to me. She was wearing denim shorts and under her skimpy white halter-top, her black bra was showing.

"My stepfather was Klan," she said. "He told me many times that if I ever brought home a nigger, he'd shoot him. At the time I didn't really agree with his views but then one day, I decided I wanted to take a florist class. It was in a school in California but I wasn't able to take the class because I didn't speak Mexican."

A few women around her shook their heads and grunted with disgust.

"That's when I realized that there was something really wrong in this country," she went on, "Now I'm the Grand Klaliff of my state."

"How old are you?" Victorine asked her.

"I'm twenty-three."

"Wow, it went really fast for you, I mean, the promotion," Victorine said.

"Yes," the woman answered with a proud look on her face.

Although I had expected to hear some racist language while working on the story, I was still shocked by her words. Remembering where I was, in the middle of a KKK picnic with people carrying guns, I made a concerted effort to hide my disgust with the mentality surrounding me and focus on gathering information. I looked at Victorine. Our eyes met in a quick but understanding glance that told me we were of like minds.

"It was the same for me," said another woman with long brunette hair that partially hid a large scar on her right cheek. She exuded an aura of toughness and seemed eager to tell her story.

"It took me several years before I decided to join the Klan. One day my car was stopped at a traffic light when a black man jumped out of the van next to me, reached in my window and grabbed my pocketbook. When I tried to grab it back he opened my door and started punchin' me. I grew up in a neighborhood where whites were a minority and constantly harassed by niggers but that was my wake-up call, when I really started to understand what was going on in this country. I worked at a university for ten years and during that time they were always pushin' their racial diversity programs down our throats: special clubs for minorities, financial aid for minorities, special classes . . . Affirmative Action."

She spat out these last words with a look of disgust on her face and the other women at the table as well as the crowd that was growing around us nodded with similar looks of disgust.

"That when I decided to take some 'Affirmative Action' of my own and joined the Klan," she said with a smirk, "but then one day, after a rally, a newspaper photographer took a photo of me without my hood. The local newspaper published it on the front page and all hell broke loose. They investigated me 'cause I was sittin' on the admissions board. They claimed I was prejudiced against black students. Then they forced me to resign."

"My son here was treated like a leper after that," she continued as put her arm around the young boy next to her who I judged to be about twelve or thirteen years old. He was tall and dark haired with vivacious eyes. "He was called a Klan baby in school and his life also became hell."

"If niggers don't bother me, I don't bother them but they're always stoppin' me on the sidewalk and tryin' to sell me crack. They all hang out in gangs, they make fun of us whites. They stink even if they take three showers a day," he said with a disgusted look on his face.

"So would you say your involvement with the Klan started with some kind of a trauma," I said, trying to use a compassionate tone as I quickly took notes.

I looked around. They were all nodding.

"I used to be a legal secretary but when they found out I was a Klan member, they fired me claiming I had too much access to people's names and personal information. Now I have to work behind the register in a gas station," said an angry voice from behind me. I turned to look. Unlike the other women around me, she was thin, pretty, and dressed smartly in tailored slacks and a simple feminine blouse. Almost elegant, she was not the image of the stereotypical redneck the KKK usually conjures up.

She repeated what has become the Klan's modern mantra, the theory supposed to make the Klan's racism more "respectable" and attract less radical members.

"You know, we don't have a problem with good black people. We have a problem with niggers. Niggers take and take from society and never give anything back. We are not Nazis. We are not a white supremacist group. We are Christian, white separatists. We don't have problems with the blacks who go to work, don't mix with drug dealers, and are productive but we have a problem with the ones who don't work, have wild parties all the time, who are stealing stuff and are destroying the neighborhood. I had a very good black friend in school, she was a good student, and she wasn't a nigger."

"That's very understandable, everybody has a problem with people who do these sorts of things," Victorine said demagogically.

"Did you gals get something to eat?" asked a huge woman wearing cut-off jeans and a Confederate flag bandana around her head.

"Well no, not yet," said Victorine, "Reverend Berry told us to help ourselves but we didn't know just who to ask."

"Oh, don't be silly, this is a picnic honey. You just come with me and I'll get you two fixed up," she said, grabbing Victorine by the arm and leading her off to one of the large buffet tables.

"Don't forget to bring something back for me," I called to Victorine as she was escorted away.

I turned to a middle-aged blonde woman sitting next to me and asked, "How about you? When did you join the Klan?"

"Well, my Mom died when I was seven and my Dad was a Klan member since I can remember. My boyfriend is also a Klan member so I decided to join too. I am not a racist as long as other races are not imposed on me. It's not about hatred, why, I even allow my eleven-year-old daughter to listen to rap music but I told her, if she ever brings a black boy home, I will disown her right away but I know that's not going to happen. She just got kicked out of school because she threw a chair at her black teacher."

Her soft voice and gentle demeanor were hard to reconcile with her harsh words.

Victorine returned with two large plates of food piled high with potato salad, beans, and two hotdogs each. The huge woman with the Confederate bandana followed her carrying another plate piled high with barbequed ribs. Victorine set down our plates, sat down opposite me, and quickly began to eat. Hungry and forbidden to take photos at this time, her interest in the stories was waning so she busied herself with her meal.

A woman, who must have been in her mid-forties, sitting to my right, had been listening quietly to the conversation. I turned to look at her and smiled. She was wearing a T-shirt that read, "You Wouldn't Understand, It's a White Thing."

"And you, would you like to share your story with us?" I asked as I picked up my fork and attempted to politely eat and listen at the same time.

She hesitated, looked around at the others and after waiting a moment she spoke.

"I've been the Grand Dragon of my state since last year. I consider myself a soldier of Christ. I am both an Aryan soldier and an Aryan mother," she said before stopping abruptly.

"Is it easy for you to be a Klan member or do you also suffer from stigmatization?" I asked.

"It is very easy for me. My six children are not part of the Klan but they support my views. I don't have any problems with them . . . with my views . . . I work as a cashier in a supermarket and very few people know I am a Klan member . . ."

She seemed anxious, in the grip of an internal conflict and finally opened up.

"Well, in fact, I do have a problem . . . with my daughter . . . Tracy. She married a black man. It may sound cruel but to me she is dead. She is not part of the family but I have no regrets. I told her I didn't want a dark illiterate bastard to call me grandma. She came one day with the baby and asked me if I wanted to see the baby. I said 'no' but I caught a glimpse of him. He was really dark," she said almost apologetically looking away with a disgusted look on her face.

Her words were greeted with an awkward silence. I put down my fork. Hearing this made me lose my appetite. I looked at the faces around the table. The woman's eyes seemed to be veiled with a deep sadness. It seemed that to them, what happened to their Klan sister was the worst kind of disaster that could befall a mother.

Victorine had finished eating. A pile of gnawed bones lay on the plate in front of her. Now ready to rejoin the conversation, she decided to lighten up the ambiance and chose the issue that was the most likely to excite the group.

"Some of you are carrying guns. Do you go through a particular training to become Grand Dragons or Grand Klaliffs?" she asked excitedly.

It worked. The women's eyes lit up. A couple of them started to speak at the same time. Laughing, they stopped in good humor. But the body guard, who had been off my radar for a while, stepped in and replied with a low-pitched drill sergeant's voice.

"Most of us have known how to use handguns since we're children but Night Hawks have to follow a special training. It lasts between three and six months. The training increases our endurance abilities. I learned how to disarm my enemies, how to shoot, target and to search people in meeting places like today. I also learned how to shoot with infrared sights at night," she said staring at me earnestly.

"Well, that's certainly very impressive. I see on your badge that you are called a 'Night Hawk.' Maybe you could tell our readers how you became a Night Hawk," I asked, realizing how proud she was of her badge.

"I was appointed Night Hawk after the ceremony of naturalization. They tested my fear, my endurance abilities. They asked me to do some physical exercise, one hundred twenty push-ups. They asked me to hunt for people in a forest, blindfolded, guided only by the sounds they made. It went well. That's how they appointed me," she said.

The other women, most of who in truth didn't look very fit, listened wide eyed, evidently in awe of her accomplishment. I noticed that our little conversation had attracted a few more onlookers.

"I've already enrolled at a white race survival camp," a young masculine-looking woman announced loudly. "It includes weapon training, guerrilla warfare, suicide teams, poison training, archery, close combat with knife and martial arts. Women learn how to give birth alone. I want to make sure I'm prepared in case the worst happens," she added eagerly.

"I can relate to that. At home, our guns are always loaded. Too often, we hear about families who got killed and burgled because their guns were not loaded," one of the new onlookers said.

At first, I wondered whether she didn't get it wrong: maybe she meant "Too often, we hear about families who get killed and burgled because their guns were loaded" but it quickly dawned on me that she meant what she said.

"And can you tell us more about the naturalization ceremony?"

"You take a sacred, secret oath of allegiance to the Klan and you become a citizen of the Klan," the bodyguard explained. "Obviously, I cannot reveal more due to my oath. But, despite the rumors, there is absolutely no blood or violence as some people may have claimed."

We passed the rest of the afternoon chatting amicably with the women. Unfortunately, Reverend Berry never returned to grant us an interview as he had promised. I noticed him pass several times, observing us. I can only guess that he received favorable reports from his security people. Even the mean-looking bodyguard relented after a while. After asking us pointed questions about the right wing party in France, she seemed satisfied, stopped monitoring us, and let us roam freely around the property. I was glad. I was getting a lot of material for our story and some of the women even revealed their names and let Victorine take photos of them (which we will not divulge out of loyalty to our sources).

As night fell, we watched the Klan members donning their robes and hoods preparing for the "cross lighting." Except for the Night Hawks wearing black and a couple of grand dragons wearing green, most members were dressed in white. We had been invited to attend the cross lighting by Reverend Berry but despite our eagerness and curiosity, seeing dozens of Klan members sneaking into the night sent shivers up my spine. The KKK costume was truly frightening and I told Victorine I wanted to leave.

"Leave!? Are you crazy? This is the reason I'm here. Where else am I going to get shots like this? Go wait in the car if you want but I'm not leaving now," she said and stomped off in a huff to look for the best vantage point

from which to photograph. She was right, so I gathered my courage, sat down on the grass, and waited. The twenty-foot cross, which had been erected in the adjacent field, had been wrapped in rags and doused with diesel fuel. At nine p.m. the participating members marched single file out onto the field carrying lit torches and formed a large circle around the cross while I stood at a safe distance, trying to contain both my fear and excitement. The young children stayed with some women in the picnic area. Reverend Berry emerged from the darkness carrying a torch. He walked briskly towards the cross and touched the flame to its base. As the cross flared, Reverend Berry stretched out his arms solemnly. Like gigantic fiery insects, the flames swiftly crawled all the way to the top and in a few seconds, the cross looked like a blazing phantom. It was a haunting sight and I found myself rooted to my spot.

"I chose to take the light of Jesus Christ. Out of the darkness comes the light. From one light come many lights, the eternal light of the KKK," Reverend Berry half shouted, half chanted as he raised and lowered his torch.

"FOR GOD!"

"FOR GOD!" All the members echoed as they raised and lowered their torches in unison. I felt a shiver go down my spine as I watched the eerily choreographed ritual.

"To the whole race!"

"To the whole race!"

"For children!"

"For children!"

"To the American Knights of the Ku Klux Klan!"

"To the American Knights of the Ku Klux Klan!"

"God bless the KKK!"

"GOD BLESS THE KKK!"

On cue, the Klan members stepped forward, threw their torches at the base of the cross then returned to their circle where they stood with their arms raised, hands joined, immobile and silent. The growing flames from the large pile of torches lit their robes with a reddish glow and the whole scene became suddenly more frightening. I sat transfixed, mesmerized by the spectral sight. The only movement was Victorine, running back and forth around the circle, shooting non-stop, trying to get the best images. The whole cross lighting ceremony lasted perhaps twenty or thirty minutes at the most and soon, as the flames died away, instead of a fiery religious symbol there stood nothing but a charred cross, threatening to crumble away. The members dispersed and I could hear them commenting on what a beautiful spectacle it had been. As I got to my feet I noticed Reverend Berry walking briskly towards me. I smiled as he approached.

"Well, Reverend Berry, we wanted to thank you for your hospitality," I said, "It was really interesting talking to the women and . . ."

"Do you know how to shoot?" he asked abruptly, interrupting me.

"Uh, I, uh, don't . . ." I stammered, searching for an answer.

Victorine appeared next to me and said, "No, we've never shot guns before."

"If you want to learn, you can attend our firearms security class tomorrow. Be here at three p.m. sharp," he said authoritatively.

"Yes, yes, we'll be here, thank you," Victorine quickly answered, probably thinking of the great photos she was going to get. We watched him turn and disappear into the darkness.

It was about 10:30 p.m. when we pulled into the campground and remembered that we still had to set up the new tent we had bought that morning. Thank goodness, the weather was good and there were no storms predicted for that night. We had completely forgotten about our kind dog sitters and were hoping they hadn't gone to sleep. They hadn't forgotten about us. A note was attached to our old crushed tent. It read:

DON'T WORRY ABOUT LOVIE. HE CAN SLEEP WITH US IN OUR MOBILE HOME TONIGHT. GOD CREATED A LOVELY LOVING DOG.

The last sentence instantly put a smile on our faces. It only took us about half an hour to figure out how to set up the new tent and by midnight we were drifting off to sleep.

I was in the middle of a bizarre dream in which snakes were crawling out of a fire and I was franticly running from a snarling dog when I was rudely awakened by barking and a recognizable strident voice.

"Oh praise the lord. It looks like they made it back safe last night," I heard Betty Jo's voice calling through our tent's thin nylon walls. "They're here sleeping in their new tent. Good morning, Natasha! Good morning, Victorine! Lovie is here. Wake up. Time to wake up!"

I struggled out of my sleeping bag and fumbled with the zipper on the tent flap. When I finally got it open I was greeted by Lovie's wet nose greeting me with doggy kisses. His tail wagging wildly, he jumped in the tent and pounced on Victorine.

"*What time is it?*" she moaned. Half asleep, she hugged Lovie and pulled him inside her sleeping bag.

I looked at my watch. It was just past seven a.m. Betty Jo's face beamed at me through the tent's opening.

"How are you two girls on this glorious God-given morning?" asked Betty Jo excitedly. "Bob is waiting for us in the car. I think you will be pleased to know that he's decided to take the three of us out for breakfast."

Victorine, hidden from Betty Jo's view behind the tent flap, looked at me wide eyed as she shook her head, silently mouthing, "No, No, No."

"Why, thank you. That's very nice of him. We'll be right with you," I answered as Victorine glared at me.

Twenty minutes later, the four of us were squeezed into a booth at the Early Bird Diner. The sun was shining through the plate glass windows, reflecting off the bright stainless steel fixtures behind the long counter.

"I'll be right back with your coffees," the waitress said as we handed her our menus.

Victorine was now happy. While Betty Jo, Bob, and I all ordered the simple breakfast special, eggs, toast, and hash browns, she had ordered the "Long-hauler's Plate": pancakes, sausage, eggs, toast, and hash browns.

"Well girls, I have good news for you," said Betty Jo, smiling. "Yes, God is good. My friend, Susie, agreed to take Lovie. She believes the good Lord put Lovie on your path to replace her lost dog. Lovie will certainly be happy with his new family. They are devoted Christians and they have a big yard."

We were both delighted and thanked Betty Jo profusely. But now it was Bob's turn and unfortunately that morning he was even more talkative than the day before.

"I know you girls are curious to know how God came to me . . ." Bob began.

"Well, we don't want to pry into your personal religious choices so . . ." Victorine started to answer, but Bob wasn't listening.

" . . . You see before I start telling you my story I want you to know that God was at work all my life but I didn't know it. I was raised a Catholic, Yes, I said prayers but I wasn't hungry for God."

Bob stopped to take a sip of his coffee.

"Oh no, here it comes. Where's that waitress with my pancakes?" said Victorine under her breath.

I pinched Victorine under the table but she avoided my eyes, maintaining her usual calm demeanor. Thankfully, they didn't understand French. Betty Jo was hanging on Bob's every word. Overwhelmed by Bob's compulsive logorrhea I sighed in despair, wondering how to escape this unbearable chatterbox. He may have been picking up the check for breakfast but we had to pay for it by listening to his sermon.

"I had an open heart surgery in October nineteen ninety-five, and wound up having more complications than I can even start to explain. Then, one day I was in my hospital bed feeling very low in a half praying and half-awake state. I was just lying there when all of a sudden I started to see a white robe with light in the corner of the ceiling and the light came in and took over the room, the light was bluish white and it moved . . ."

Thankfully, the waitress arrived with our order and I expected Bob to take a break and eat his breakfast but Bob just looked at us eagerly. I widened my eyes and feigned extreme curiosity. Satisfied by my inquisitive expression, he continued with his story while his eggs grew cold.

"I remembered thinking I was dreaming but the intensity was so great I thought I was leaving my body going towards the light. And as I said, the light was moving and hair appeared coming to me, golden hair with a face and He was coming to me with this light, his palms were facing me and his hands were down. He came to me and I was electrified. I knew what it was. I asked Him to forgive me and told Him I loved Him. When I finished saying that I knew it wasn't a dream and I was in tears . . ."

Bob started to cry and a cascade of tears trickled onto his toast. Betty Jo quickly handed him a napkin to dry his eyes and put her arm around his shoulders to comfort him. This man was just too much with the drama. I thought that I was going to cry too if this torture didn't finish soon. As Bob composed himself I looked over at Victorine. Her pancakes were gone and she was busy spreading butter on her toast.

"Pass the salt," she said to me.

"Can't you even be polite and listen?" I said through clenched teeth as I handed her the saltshaker.

"I am polite. Just smile, nod your head and eat your breakfast before it gets cold," she said, *"Trust me, he just loves to hear himself talk . . . watch."*

Victorine looked at Bob and Betty Jo and gave them a sweet smile and an understanding nod.

"What happened then, Bob?" she asked as she sprinkled salt on her eggs.

Bob smiled back and continued with his story. As usual Victorine was right.

"Well, it was at that point he said, 'you come to me you will be saved.' It was evidently a full-blown vision of Jesus Chris. Jesus assured me that He will lead me to people who worship Him in Spirit. I wouldn't trade that experience for anything in this world. It's the power of the Spirit of GOD Almighty. God will totally change you if you accept him. I encourage you to try JESUS CHRIST because He is a powerful God. Ask Jesus to show Himself to you and pray for it, and He will give the desire of your heart according to His will. God, it was a remarkable experience that I will never forget. Praise the Lord, Amen, Halleluiah."

"Well, that's quite a story, Bob. What do you think, Natasha?" Victorine asked as she held up her coffee cup, signaling to the waitress for a refill.

"Mmhmm . . . Pretty amazing . . ." I said with a mouthful of hash browns.

"See, I told you girls," Betty Jo said excitedly.

But Bob wasn't finished.

"So, you see girls, I am sharing my testimony with you so that one day you could be open to God and when He comes to you, you will know you will be saved and loved until your dying days. Because God loves you, He even loves those that are unlovable, He knows how to walk with someone that betrays him and still can love them regardless. Thank You Jesus for being our mighty God. Both the Lion and the Lamb . . ."

Bob's unsolicited sermon was beginning to really annoy me. I decided to interrupt him as diplomatically as I could.

"Yes, that's very true, Bob, very true and enlightening," I said as I grabbed my purse and slid out of the booth. "Thank you for sharing your amazing testimony with us. But I think we need to get back to the campground now and prepare for this afternoon's interview. Thank you for helping to find a lovely home for Lovie. We'll walk back to the campground. The fresh air will do us good."

Bob and Betty Jo seemed a little disappointed as we waved goodbye and practically flew out of the diner, just in time too because we both exploded with laughter the minute we got outside. We laughed all the way as we walked back to the campground. Luckily it took my mind off our dreaded upcoming meeting with Reverend Berry.

As instructed, we arrived at Reverend Berry's at exactly three p.m. Again we were searched, this time a bit less thoroughly, by the same security guard as the day before. We were then instructed to follow a dirt path down to the shooting range. My trepidation grew as we walked through the woods and the sound of gunshots grew louder and louder. The path opened into a lovely isolated clearing next to a river at the far corner of the compound. Approximately thirty Klan members were attending what Reverend Berry called his "firearm security class." About ten people, half of them women, were lined up in a row, shooting all kinds of hand guns and rifles at paper targets tacked to boards against an earthen embankment on the far side of the clearing. All were wearing large headsets over their ears, the kind you see worn by aircraft maintenance workers on the tarmac at airports. The gunshots were making a terrifying racket and I was contemplating turning to leave when our friend the female security guard spotted us and waved us to come join her.

"Vicky! Natasha!" she yelled excitedly over the din of the gunshots, "Come join me over here. I'll show you how to shoot!"

There was no way I could decline. I knew she wanted to share her passion with us and meant well. I also knew that the experience of two French girls taking gun-shooting classes with the KKK would be a salient part of the reportage. She handed us each a headset. We put them on and I immediately felt a bit more comfortable. At least I could hear myself think now that the ear-splitting noise was dampened a bit.

"This is a Beretta revolver. Here's the safety . . . now it's on . . . now it's off. First you have to acquire your target; then get into a nice aggressive stance. Your arms have to be out . . ." she said, bending at the knees and elbows slightly and cradling the revolver with two hands pointing at the target.

From the corner of my eye I noticed Reverend Berry studying us but I kept my attention on our instructor. I had never even been this close to a gun before, let alone shot one, and I didn't want to miss a thing lest I wind up shooting off one of my toes.

"To hold a gun correctly, you want your hips and shoulders square to the target. Don't move your shoulders, relax your arms and look at the target. You got it?"

Victorine nodded assuredly. I managed a nod too but I think it was more of a tremble.

"The left hand is your support arm, it must be under the gun, and your fingers along the bottom trigger guard so it encompasses the entire side of the gun. The front side should be in line with the tip of the elbow and you have to make contact with both hands on the four corners of the gun," she said, cradling the gun with her two hands.

"Once you have a firm grip, you squeeze the trigger."

BANG! The gun fired and I jumped. My heart was racing. Even with the headset it was a deafening sound. Her arm shook a little as she fired.

"I've been shooting for almost twenty years," said the man next to us on the firing line. He had a ponytail, long grey beard, and dressed like he rode Harley-Davidson motorcycles.

"The nine millimeter kicks less, it has a lot less flips, and it holds a couple more rounds than the forty-five which enables you to shoot better."

I smiled and nodded but had no idea what he was talking about. I'm not even sure I heard him correctly. He might as well have been speaking Chinese to me.

"Do you want to try?" our instructor asked.

"I'll try," Victorine said eagerly. I declined politely.

Our instructor carefully handed the gun to Victorine. As instructed she bent slightly at her knees, held out her arms, cradled the handgun and BANG! The shot projected her backward slightly but her cheeks were red and her eyes were wide with excitement.

"Excellent, Vicky!" our instructor exclaimed, turning to me with an expectant look.

"*Natasha, you really have to try it!*" Victorine said to me, then our instructor, "I had no idea the shot could shake your body so much! It's like an explosion!"

"Oh, no . . . First, I don't like explosions. Second, I'm not so strong. It might put me flat on my butt!"

I was trying to joke my way out of the situation but there was no countering Victorine's determined pleas, which in fact were more and more like orders. Once again, I felt frightened like a cornered doe but I had to put on a brave front. There I stood, trembling, with my arms outstretched and my heart pounding, trying to remember all the instructions. I tried to get a firm grip on my revolver and slowly, but not so surely, I squeezed the trigger and BANG! I jumped like a frightened cat, my eyes widened with fear and my mouth twisted. Petrified, I stayed immobile for a few seconds.

"That's . . . that' it. I've . . . I've done it . . ." I said, my arms still stretched as if I was going to shoot again.

Victorine laughed. I must have looked comical.

"Very good, girls! You're welcome to try again."

"*Isn't it something?*" Victorine asked excitedly.

"*Yes, but once is enough for me,*" I said carefully handing her the gun.

Of course, Victorine hadn't had enough and continued shooting. Prudently, I decided to retreat to the rear of the firing line, away from all that crazy noise, where I stood and watched Victorine and the other shooters. As I gradually regained my composure I thought about the events of the last two days, organizing the material in my head. It had been truly enlightening. In truth, the KKK women didn't seem particularly evil. Maybe more misguided than anything else. It dawned on me that these women's stories were far more complex than just hatred. Their chaotic family histories seemed to suggest that they were still mostly searching for a sense of belonging, which they had found in their extended KKK family, and that in some bizarre way, they might also have been the uncomprehending victims of some perverse twists of fate. Who knows where any of us would wind up if our life's circumstances were different?

During our two days with the Klan, we didn't have many interactions with Reverend Berry. He remained somewhat of a mysterious figure to us but we were thankful that we had obeyed his strict rules. We later learned to our amazement, that after our encounter he served three years of a seven-year sentence for sequestering two journalists and holding them at gunpoint. We also learned that about a year after we met him he was involved in a violent fight with his son. The assault left him in critical condition with a swollen brain stem. Doctors gave him only a 50 percent chance of survival and said that even if Berry lived, his life would never be the same. Before being sent to prison, Berry was the national leader of the American Knights of the Ku Klux Klan. At the time, the group was known as the largest and most aggressive Klan faction in America, with twenty-seven chapters in 2000. Today, the American Knights of the Ku Klux Klan is defunct.

Grandma's Ambrosia Salad

- 2 oranges
- ½ teaspoon orange peel, grated
- 1 cup coconut, fresh frozen or shredded fresh preferably
- 2 ounces fresh pineapple or 1 can pineapple
- 2 apples, diced
- ¼ cup brown sugar

1. Drain pineapple, saving ¼ cup juice in a small saucepan.
2. Add brown sugar and orange peel to the pineapple juice, heat until sugar dissolves.
3. Peel and dice the oranges, removing all white pith and pits.
4. In individual parfait glasses or fruit bowl, arrange orange, apple, and pineapple.
5. Add pineapple juice mixture and stir gently.
6. Chill about 1 hour.
7. Add coconut right before serving.

Mousse au Chocolat (Chocolate Mousse)
Serves 6 to 8

- 10 ounces semi sweet chocolate
- 6 eggs (preferably organic)
- ½ lemon, juiced

1. Separate the egg yolks from whites.
2. In a small sauce pan, melt the chocolate using the bain-marie technique, stirring nonstop with a wooden spoon until smooth.
3. When the chocolate has cooled down a little, add the egg yolks, one by one and mix well.
4. Beat your egg whites with an electric mixer until frothy and hard (to test, turn the bowl upside down and the whites should not fall down).
5. Gently incorporate the chocolate to the egg whites.
6. Add the lemon juice.
7. Pour the mousse into individual ramequins or a big bowl and chill for 2 to 3 hours.

Chapter Ten

Les Misérables

W e awoke early the next morning, packed the car and drove all the next day. I was glad to get away from the noisy guns and see the lit-up pinnacle of the Empire State Building beckon us as we entered New York City late that night. Compared to the places we had seen, New York City symbolized Enlightenment to me. Unlike Victorine, I didn't have an insatiable thirst for adventure. I was proud of our reportage and felt we had done some great stories, some of which had made newspapers' front pages. My self-confidence was finally returning after the ego-shattering experience of my academic failure. All I wanted now was a little break from the excitement and to maybe cover some more "conservative" stories that wouldn't make my adrenaline sky-rocket. This is how, after noticing the increasing numbers of can collectors in New York City, we ended up on the corner of Third Avenue and Eighty-first Street interviewing James, a disheveled thirty-nine-year-old man dressed in stained denim jeans and a navy blue sweatshirt. James spent his days relentlessly rummaging through tons of garbage on New York City's streets, searching for glass and metal cans. We spent the better part of a day speaking with him as he frantically pushed his overflowing shopping cart in and out of the impatient honking city traffic. I realized how true the saying was, "One man's trash is another's treasure." Seeing the city from this point of view was eye opening and really, the amount of soda cans and bottles left on the street was shocking.

"People don't bother redeemin' their cans so I do it for them," said James, "I get five cents for each can or bottle. I work six days a week from nine a.m. to six p.m. and I make about fifty dollars a day."

I quickly calculated that James had to collect one thousand cans to earn fifty dollars a day. What a grueling job. I was amazed. On top of everything, he was an environmentalist, fortuitous indeed, but still, society seemed to rely on him to recover and salvage its refuse.

"I'm impressed, James. You're homeless but you work harder than most people I know," I said. He turned quickly and glared at me.

"I'm not homeless," he said indignantly, "I work all day, then I go home, relax, and watch TV in my room."

"Wow, you manage to pay for your own room by picking up garbage?" said Victorine, who was now also glaring at me in admonishment for my insult.

"I live in a free room in the tunnel under the subway," James answered proudly as he went back to sorting his metal and glass.

Victorine and I looked at each other then back at James. Did we hear him correctly?

"A room . . . under . . . the subway?" Victorine asked dubiously.

"Yeah, a lot of us do. We're mole people," he said nonchalantly, "If you want I'll take you down there. You'll see. There's a whole city livin' under the streets."

James' words made Victorine's photographic antennae vibrate frantically.

"James, where can we find you tomorrow? We'd like to ask you a few more questions for our article," asked Victorine.

"Well, I usually make my rounds and wind up at the D'Agostinos on Lexington and Eighty-Third, somewhere between six and seven," he answered as he rummaged through a waste bin, pulling out two Coke cans.

"Look for us, we'll be around," she said.

"James, thank you for taking the time to speak to us today. I'm sure we slowed you down a bit today and you probably lost some money because of us, so please take this to help make up for any time from work you lost," I said as I pressed a neatly folded twenty-dollar bill into his palm.

James looked at his palm, then at both of us with a smile as he slid the bill into his pocket.

"Anytime ladies. I'm happy to help, happy to help. I'll look for you tomorrow," he said.

We watched him walk away, wheeling his cart down the sidewalk, stopping at the next trash bin to check for cans. When he turned the corner Victorine started repeating, "Mole people, mole people, mole people . . . *Natasha, I've heard that before . . . Wait! I think I've heard of a book about them. Come on.*"

She grabbed my arm and dragged me down the crowded sidewalk, ignoring the curses of the elegant Upper East Siders we bumped into as we raced to the Eighty-Sixth Street Border's Booksellers.

"Don't you realize? If that guy is right, we have the story of our lifetime. It's like discovering a whole community living in the Parisian Catacombs," Victorine said, evidently thrilled by the idea of getting into some kind of new frightening adventure.

I was convinced that James was a fantasist but she, as usual, had a completely different take on the situation.

"Mole people . . . the mole people," the hollow-cheeked sales clerk murmured under his breath as looked up the title on the store's database, "Ah yes, here it is," he said squinting at the screen, "*The Mole People* by Jennifer Toth, 1993 . . . and we have one left in stock, follow me."

We followed him to the other side of the store where he found the book in the racks and handed it to Victorine. She gazed at the cover wide eyed then turned it around and held it up victoriously for me to see. THE MOLE PEOPLE: LIFE IN THE TUNNELS BENEATH NEW YORK CITY. The cover showed a black and white photo of a tunnel lit up by light streaming through an open manhole.

"We've got to talk to these people. Imagine the photos I'm going to get." Victorine whispered excitedly.

That's how our "mole people story" began. That night, as Victorine devoured her new book, I woke up screaming and sweating, frightened by a horrible nightmare: a gigantic creature, half mole, half man, was chasing me through an underground labyrinth. I woke up at the very moment I slipped on a Coke bottle and the mole was about to pounce on me. It certainly wasn't a good start. The damn story was already affecting me and I had a hard time getting back to sleep. Over next morning's breakfast Victorine read from sections of the book she had highlighted.

"Listen to this," she said, "In nineteen hundred, the city of New York began construction of the most expansive underground railway system in the world. By 1940 there was a maze of subway tunnels over seven hundred and forty miles long under the city's streets. By the end of the twentieth century, many tunnels and stations became obsolete and were forgotten, . . . *you see, that obviously must be where the mole people are hiding . . . Imagine if there was a whole secret city down there with a mayor and . . ."*

"OK, enough, listen I have to finish my story on can collectors," I said.

As I sat trying to write, I could hear Victorine in the next room calling homeless organizations for information about the mole people. Convinced that all this agitation was futile and that mole people were just an urban myth, I tried to ignore her. Two hours later she appeared in the doorway with notebook in hand and a triumphant smile.

"Listen, I think we have our story," she said as she scanned her notes, *"According to a study made by New York City's Department of Health and Mental Hygiene, 6,031 homeless people were living under Grand Central and Penn stations in 1991. New York authorities say that the numbers decreased greatly after the Amtrak clean-up program under Grand Central station in 1995, but, according to charitable organizations, there's probably a few thousand people still living in the tunnels. Where else would all these people be? They have to be somewhere, right?"*

"Okay, just suppose there ARE people living down there," I said irritably, *"How are you going to meet them? I suppose you're planning to go down there alone with your little flashlight?"*

"Don't you remember what James said? When we meet him this eve-ning, we'll see if we can trust him and ask him to take us down there," she answered self-confidently.

Everything was so simple for Victorine. Should I tell her about my terrifying nightmare? I was about to but stopped short. I knew she would just belittle me for being scared, the same way she did when we were young and I refused to ride her spirited stallion. *"What a chicken you are!"* she would say. I decided to keep silent. There was still a chance that James was just spreading an urban myth and had no intention of bringing us down below the streets. Unfortunately for me, James kept his word and we found him outside D'Agostinos, redeeming three huge blue bags full of cans. He greeted us with a bright smile and an hour later, the three of us were sitting inside a nearby McDonald's, devouring double cheeseburgers. Victorine, anxious to get information, started the questions.

"So James, how long have you been living under the streets?"

James looked up, his eyes quickly scanned the surrounding tables, then he leaned closer.

"I've been livin' in the tunnel for about six years now," he answered, "The tunnel is my home, my first real home ever. I live down there and I work up here."

"But isn't it dangerous down there?" she asked.

"Are you kiddin'?" he responded incredulously, "I only feel safe when I'm down there. I have my protection down there. Listen, one time before I found my place in the tunnel, I was sleepin' on a bench in a park when I got woken up by a bunch of teenagers. They were kickin' me, pourin' lighter fluid on me and trying to set my clothes on fire . . . but I was ready. I always sleep with my baseball bat and I just started swingin' it, actin' all crazy. I broke one of those little bastard's knee-caps and those other chicken-shits just ran. No, no, no, I prefer to stay underground where it's safe."

"You wouldn't prefer to go to a shelter?" I asked.

"Have you ever spent the night in a shelter?" he asked, fixing me with a gaze that made me feel embarrassed for asking the question. I shook my head, "No."

"Shelters are worse than the street," he said with disgust, "The second you turn your back or go to sleep, someone steals your stuff. They're not safe, plus there's too many rules. It's like jail there, man."

"Do many tunnel inhabitants take drugs?" I asked cautiously.

"Yeah, most I know but the cops don't bother them there. It's our territory. The cops are scared of us and they're scared of the third rail. People get electrocuted by the third rail. When the train's coming, its lights blind you and it's easy to trip and fall."

I was dying to ask James whether he had a prison history but it seemed too early.

"Are any of the tunnel inhabitants criminals?" I finally ventured, ill prepared for what was to come.

"Yeah, most of the people I know have been in jail. I was in for seventeen years for armed burglary. I spent time in all the New York prisons. It used to be you could study and take exams in jail but not no more. When I got out I filed for a public housing apartment but they wouldn't give it to me 'cause I had a police record. I really wanted to leave the past behind me but I finally understood that this society is going to do everything it can to crush me," said James somewhat aggressively.

"*That's enough for tonight, let's go. We'll continue tomorrow,*" I said softly yet firmly to Victorine. She nodded in agreement and after arranging another rendezvous the next evening we left James as he packed up our leftover fries into a takeout box.

"*You must be out of your mind! There's no way I'm going down there with a guy who spent seventeen years in jail!*" I yelled at Victorine once we were outside on the crowded sidewalk.

"*Okay, okay,*" she answered calmly.

James' prison history made me excessively uncomfortable and without Victorine, I would certainly have broken off all relations with him and given up on the mole story. I guess she was quicker than me to detect his humanity under the layers of hurt and trauma which had turned him into a heroin addict. She wanted to go deeper. I knew then that it had less to do with the photographs she could take than with her humanism. That night as I lay in bed drifting off to sleep, I suddenly sat bolt upright, wide awake.

A realization came to me all at once. I remembered our final evening in Texas, which now seemed a lifetime ago, and the horrible scene with our two racist Texans, Lynn and Jack. Their words rang in my head ..."crime is in their blood." I felt sick to my stomach again but this time it was because I realized the way I was acting was no better than either of them. What right did I have to judge James? Who knows where any of us could wind up if our life's circumstances were different? I grew up on an idyllic horse farm in the pastoral French countryside with two loving parents who nurtured and encouraged me. Any twist of fate could have landed me in a far different situation, one where I might have had to fight just to survive. I resolved myself to not judge James and learn his story.

Every evening that week, we treated James to a McDonald's cheeseburger and fries. It was clearly an unusual event for him.

"I rarely buy my own food. What's the point?" he said. "People throw away so much good food. I salvage it."

I sensed he felt more and more comfortable in our presence as he opened up and told us about his past. Perhaps he was looking for acknowledgement from people besides those in his same circumstances. I had noticed during my brief time living in New York that the homeless were invisible to most people as they go about their day on the bustling city streets. By the end of the week I was captivated by the story of his traumatic life.

"My stepfather used to beat the shit out of us and my mom never lifted a finger to defend us. I couldn't take it anymore so I grabbed his wallet one night when he was sleepin' and just left. I was about fourteen then. I slept in abandoned houses, buildings, any place I could find. You know just livin' on the street, hustlin', whatever I had to do to get by. Then I started huffin'."

We must have had blank stares of non-comprehension because he looked at both of us then explained.

"Huffin' . . . you know, sniffin' glue, one of my friends said, 'Here try this it will make you feel better,' and it did, anythin' to make you numb, to make you forget. Then, I tried H, just sniffin' it at first. I was scared to start shootin' up at first but then I did and then after a while it was anything to get a fix . . . anything, anything," he repeated as his eyes locked with mine in a penetrating stare that told me that even my imagination couldn't conjure up the depths some people reach out of desperation.

"I started stealin', you know, smash and grab, handbags, whatever, then, I got stupid. Me and a friend got a gun and we started robbin' people. First it was stores, then people's apartments. It was bad. A lot of it I don't even remember but it comes back to me in flashes, you know, like I'm watchin' it on TV but it's like, I know it's me. I promised myself I was going to get out of it. That's why I'm enrolled in the methadone program to stop takin' heroin. I'm clean now. I go to the treatment center every day," James said proudly as he showed us his syringe-scarred forearms.

"It is hard goin' through life with no one at all. No family, no friends, no one who gives a damn. The streets take away all your confidence. You have to build up that confidence again from scratch. Believe me, I know it's not the best place to live but the security of the tunnel helps me now. I will make it out of there one day," James said in a vulnerable, quivering voice filled with honesty.

We were moved. At the age of thirty-nine, James had the courage to leave his criminal past behind him and to fight social standards that branded him as an unredeemable social pariah. His words conjured up Victor Hugo's Jean Valjean in *Les Misérables*. Where did he find the hope after suffering so much injustice? In his quest for emotional survival, it seemed that the tunnel was James' best friend.

After weeks of field research at the Bowery shelter center, interviewing homeless people, we finally discovered some current and former "mole people." They all had the same sorrowful look in their eyes, of people who had "crossed to the other place" where life and death get so close that they became almost undistinguishable. They each had found solace and safety in the tunnel. We became acutely aware of two oppositional universes surrounding us. We couldn't walk on New York City's streets without thinking about the world below our feet that was a distorted reflection of the one above. Threatening, inhabited by dark souls, it seemed to me that it was the embodiment of the irrational and the unconscious as if in some way, New York had buried in its entrails its darkest part, its human refuse, people who felt so undesirable that they preferred to hide. We were about to visit the world of the mole people and James would be our guide.

Early one morning the following week we went with James to Grand Central Terminal. As a precaution we brought our friend Natalie along who we asked to wait for us at the coffee shop with instructions to call the police if we weren't back in one hour. That seemed like enough time since I didn't want to venture too far into the tunnels. I mostly wanted to see James' "home" and, if possible, a few other homes. Armed with our backpacks, flashlights, and hiking shoes, we set off to explore New York City's tunnels. We followed him down the stairs, and through the turnstiles to the end of the platform of the number six train where we stopped at a yellow gate with a sign that read "DO NOT ENTER OR CROSS TRACKS." A train was just entering the station.

"We wait for everyone to board the train," he called to us over the rumble, "and as soon as it leaves you follow me over the railing and stay close to the wall. Don't worry, the cops won't catch us."

"What happens if they do?" I asked.

"They'll arrest us for criminal trespassing."

"Criminal trespassing?" I repeated. Foolishly I had forgotten that what we were doing was illegal. I didn't know what would happen if the police caught us but I figured that like in Paris, our press pass would quickly calm them down. I was wrong of course. New York City police didn't care about two crazy French reporters. I was starting to have misgivings about this whole adventure but it was too late, people had boarded the train and it was leaving the station.

"Come on, stay close to me," James said as the train rumbled away.

We quickly climbed over the railing and followed him along a narrow side ledge that ran against the wall about a hundred feet. At the end we climbed down a little ladder leading to the tracks. My stomach was in knots. I peered down the darkened tunnel. A string of small white lights strung overhead trailed off into the blackness. Off in the distance I heard a low rumble punctuated by odd grinding and metallic squeaks and squeals which seemed to be coming from all directions.

"Okay, we're good. Now, the first thing, see that?" James said, pointing to a large raised rail running along the side of the tracks, "That's the third rail. Be very, very careful and make sure you don't step on it. It supplies the electricity that runs the trains. Seven hundred and fifty volts. If you touch it you'll be fried instantly."

Victorine and I nodded in unison. She was unusually quiet, a sure sign that she was as nervous as I.

"Remember," James continued, "If a train comes you need to get off the tracks fast. They come quicker than you think so always keep your eyes open for a place to hide. Okay, now follow me."

My heart raced and my hands were shaking. I followed Victorine and James along the tracks, lighting the ground ahead of me with my flashlight. I tried to stay calm using the deep steady breathing exercises I had learned in my yoga classes but the air in the tunnel was quite foul. The odor of old rotting garbage and urine filled my nostrils and I found it easier to take shallow breaths through my mouth. I was nervous but determined to see James' home. Ahead of us, it was really dark but I could make out that the tunnel had opened up to a larger space. We stepped up onto a little platform where a vaulted wall was covered with black graffiti. My eyes were getting used to the darkness but soon the whitish lights gave way to bluish lights that made the atmosphere truly alienating. It felt like we were on another planet. Suddenly we heard the rumbling noise and the lights of a train approaching.

"Stand in between those pillars!" James yelled.

Victorine grabbed my hand and squeezed it so hard I thought my bones were going to break. My heart was pounding. We both carefully stepped over the third rail and flattened ourselves against the wall between two pillars. Dazzled by the approaching lights, I closed my eyes and waited anxiously. The train, pushing the air ahead of it in the narrow tunnel, created a wind that sent dust and debris swirling up all around us. I buried my nose in the sleeve of my jacket and gasped for air. Now we were standing a foot or so away from the passing train's metal wheels clattering on the rails. The sound was deafening. Calm yourself, calm yourself, I kept repeating to myself. It seemed like an eternity but the train finally passed and we crept out of our hiding place. Ever careful of the third rail we continued following James down the tracks. Slowly my heartbeat returned to normal.

"Watch out, track rabbits!" James called over his shoulder with a laugh as two gray shadows slipped between Victorine's feet. I jumped aside, pointed my flashlight at the shadows, and the beam revealed two enormous rats scurrying down the tracks.

"Ahhh!" she shrieked in terror, jumping aside. I also jumped but Victorine's reaction was so comical that I had to laugh. I had forgotten that Victorine had always been terrified of rats. Although a devoted animal lover, rats and mice were her one phobia for which she had no explanation. Even as a child the tiny French mice in our Papa's barn would send her up the walls so these "track rabbits" might traumatize her for life. Still, she marched on bravely but I could tell from her rigid stance and her lowered head that she was now petrified. The blue lights were behind us and track ahead was strung with more white lights. James shined his flashlight on a large walled up area ahead. My eyes were now accustomed to the darkness and I could make out a ladder leading up to what looked like an enclosed space.

"Somebody lives here. It's a bunker," he said.

I felt the ground shake, heard another rumbling, and saw lights bouncing off the walls. My stomach tightened and I froze as my eyes searched for the nearest hiding place.

"Don't worry, that train's on the other track," said James as he went on walking towards the bunker.

"Yo! Anybody there?" he called as he climbed up the short ladder into the bunker. There was no answer. Victorine and I climbed in behind him. Bunkers are the concrete rooms where MTA employees took their work breaks. The "home" consisted of a filthy mattress and a wooden crate, now functioning as a nightstand, with a kerosene lamp on it. Piles of dirty clothes were scattered around the room as well as beer bottles and other trash. It wasn't the structured environment we had envisioned. Victorine pulled her camera from her backpack and took a couple of quick photos before we left.

"Come on, Diego's waitin'," said James climbing down the ladder. He continued resolutely down the track, and I froze and turned to look at Victorine.

"*What did he say?*" I asked excitedly.

"*I don't know, that sounded weird but let's go. I don't want to lose him and get lost down here,*" she said pulling me ahead by the arm.

We followed James along the tracks to another bunker. As he climbed the ladder he called out, "Hey man, I'm back. They're with me now, you cool?"

I heard a muffled grunt from inside.

"Welcome to my home!" said James with a huge smile as he motioned to us to enter. The room was more spartan than I expected. On one side lay an empty mattress and on the other lay another mattress with a pale unhealthy looking Hispanic man in his mid-thirties, sitting drinking a beer.

"This is Diego," said James, then he turned to Diego and said, "these are the ones I was telling you about, Natasha and Victorine."

Diego didn't move but looked up at us through bleary unfocused eyes.

"Natash 'n Victory, Natash 'n Victory," he repeated.

Empty cans, bottles and food wrappers lay strewn around and on Diego's mattress. He made an effort to stand but fell back down, ignoring the beer which spilled all over him. A candle sat burning in a hardened pool of melted wax on the milk crate next to him and even in the minimal light I could see his state was more than just drunk or sick.

"You see, I've got everything here," James explained excitedly trying to get my attention, "To wash, I get water from the fire hydrants. There's a lot of water down here. So I wash from head to toe. It's really important to be clean. Otherwise you'd go crazy."

"Didn't you tell me you had a TV?" I asked, looking around.

"Well, yeah, uh, that was, that was in my other place," James stammered, his eyes avoiding mine, "but we traded that for, well, for some other stuff. I don't have time to watch TV now."

A distinct odor of urine permeated the air. Victorine quickly took several photos of James and Diego, the overall room, the dirty mattresses and the meager furnishings. We then climbed down the ladder and started back toward the train platform.

"You're sure you don't want to go on exploring?" asked James as he followed us out.

"No, I don't want to get arrested by the police," said Victorine flatly.

"James, who is Diego?" I asked.

"I told you about him, he's my protection," said James.

"Protection? He protects you?" I asked.

"My space, my space . . . my home," answered James loudly and aggressively, "I can't leave my space and my stuff here while I'm up top. Diego protects my space, makes sure no one messes with my stuff and I take care of what he needs."

"And what does he need?" I asked, but the entire scenario was becoming clear to me. I had a good idea of the answer. Having a home anywhere has its price and I learned that James was a "runner" which in the world of the mole people was someone who ventures up top to get essentials for living. Diego was a "sitter" or "protection," the person who stays below, rarely venturing above ground, protecting the precious underground real estate from intrusion or theft. It was a bizarre symbiotic relationship born out of necessity and I had a strong suspicion that a large chunk of the money James was earning from his can and bottle collecting was going towards drugs for Diego.

"*I've seen enough. Come on, let's get out of here,*" said Victorine nervously tugging on my arm. I could tell by the tightness in her voice she was scared. I could understand. The whole experience was quite unnerving but, for the first time in our lives, she was more scared than I. It had the odd effect of making me feel confident and a bit more relaxed. We thanked James and made our way back without incident to the coffee shop at Grand Central Terminal to report to Natalie. Truth be told, I was as relieved as Victorine to get outside into the sunshine. Our expedition had lasted just over an hour and although we hadn't seen the underground city described by Jennifer Toth, we did have our first concrete evidence that mole people truly existed. Still, to make our story truly compelling we needed some more examples. During our investigations we had met other people who claimed they lived in the tunnels. One of them was Brooklyn, a forty-year-old woman who told us she lived below Riverside Park in the Amtrak tunnel that was built in the 1930s. She had given us her "address" and we were scheduled to meet her in the afternoon at 112th Street and Riverside Drive. As we headed uptown on the subway Victorine and I sat silently in our seats, our eyes glued to the darkness beyond the glass, peering into the world of which we had heretofore been oblivious.

We found Brooklyn sitting on a bench near the park entrance stuffing bags into an old collapsible shopping cart. It was a sunny autumn day and the air was a bit brisk but she was dressed in a heavy winter coat, hat, and boots. As we got closer I saw that the coat was covering many layers of shirts and sweaters underneath. A wool skirt covered torn gray sweat pants.

"I didn't think you two were gonna show up," was her only greeting.

"We're glad we did and we want to thank you for agreeing to show us your home," I said.

"Yes, thank you," said Victorine, "and we'd like to offer you something for your time and trouble."

Victorine stepped closer and discreetly offered Brooklyn a folded ten-dollar bill. She looked at it, then warily to her left and right before taking it.

"Yeah, well I AM busy but I'm happy to help you two with your story," she said.

We followed her through the park then off the designated sidewalk onto a dirt path that led to a concealed opening in the bushes. The path ended at a concrete wall with a rusted metal door. The bottom of the door was rusted through and beneath it the dirt was dug out leaving enough space for a person to squeeze through.

"Watch your head," she warned us as she crawled inside, dragging her cart behind her.

Victorine and I looked at each other.

"After you," I said, gesturing with a courtly bow.

"Oh no, no, after you my dear," she replied, bowing in return.

"*Please, I insist,*" I said switching on my flashlight and shining it into the dark opening.

Defeated, Victorine cradled her camera protectively in her arms and squeezed under the door into the darkness. Once we were both inside and my eyes adjusted to the darkness I was surprised to see that this Amtrak tunnel was a much larger and more hospitable place than the MTA tunnel under Grand Central Terminal. Two tracks ran side by side and the high vaulted ceiling and sturdy-looking structures felt more protective than claustrophobic.

"They don't use these tracks regular no more," said Brooklyn, "you only see a train once in a while. Come on, my place is up here."

Daylight shone through large grates overhead, revealing violent graffiti on the concrete walls. The scent of fresh air floated down from above. We followed as Brooklyn pulled her cart along the tracks then veered off to the left and into the shadows. I switched on my flashlight, pointed its beam into the darkness ahead and was startled to see about half a dozen sets of feline eyes peering back at me.

"Welcome to my home. These are my babies . . . all waiting for dinner, aren't cha. You waitin' for Momma, aren't cha," she said as cats came running out of the darkness, rubbed up against her legs and sniffed at her cart. She pulled aside a large piece of plywood that camouflaged an opening in the wall and motioned us to step inside a protected alcove that looked like it might once have been a tool storage area. The cats followed us and we were welcomed by more already inside.

One corner of the dirt floor in the twelve by twelve–foot room was strewn with empty tuna cans and chicken bones. In the opposite corner a nest of candles sat on a wooden crate next to a mattress that was elevated on two shipping palettes. The odor of old tuna and cat urine filled the air. I went back to breathing shallowly through my mouth.

Brooklyn sat on her mattress and invited us to sit down on two milk crates across from her as she lit the candles next to her. About a dozen cats meowed hungrily and one jumped in my lap.

Brooklyn laughed, "I calls him Donald Trump 'cause he looks like he's wearin' a smokin' jacket."

Another cat lay down next to her and rolled on his back demanding to be pet. She smiled and obliged.

"Do you mind if I take a few pictures of you and your babies?" asked Victorine.

"No, you go right ahead. They'll all be here now 'cause they know it's time for supper," said Brooklyn as she pulled bags out of her cart, unwrapped what looked like discarded tidbits of food and tossed them in the corner. The cats all pounced on them, hissing and fighting over their individual shares.

"I wouldn't sit down on anything if I were you. Who knows how many fleas are in here," Victorine said to me as she smiled at Brooklyn.

This sudden realization hit me and I stiffened, then gently lifted and placed Donald Trump down on the floor with his friends. Trying not to think about the thousands of fleas who were making my socks their new home I asked Brooklyn, "So, how long have you been here?"

"Oh, I've been livin' here, takin' care of my 'babies' in this 'igloo' since 1982, ever since my parents died and our house was set on fire. This is my refuge against human meanness."

"How did you find this place?" I asked.

"I didn't find it. Oh no, no, no," said Brooklyn emphatically, then leaning forward and looking at me intently she continued, "I was brought here. Mmm, hmm, that's right. After I lost my house I didn't have no place to go and I was sleeping on a bench in the park by the river. This cat right, Hudson I called him, well, Hudson came to see me. He was just sittin' there, lookin' at me and meowin' . . . you know, meow, meow, meow . . . just like that. Then he come up and sits in my lap. He stayed for a long time and we becomes friends, then he jumps down and starts looking at me and meowin' again, meow, meow, meow . . . just like that. Well, I follows him and he brings me right here, right HERE . . . to my new house."

"A cat, Hudson . . . brought you here?" I asked.

"That's right. He brought me here to take care of him and his friends," Brooklyn said as she pulled more scraps of food from another bag and tossed them to the crowd of cats in the corner.

Our visit ended when Brooklyn told us that she had to go to do some more "dumpster diving." Victorine was packing up her camera and I could tell by the disgusted look on her face that she had seen enough.

"My babies have eaten. Now it's time for me to find something to eat," she said.

We followed her back to the street, thanked her and said goodbye. Victorine had seen enough and I was relieved, thinking we had no more feats to accomplish.

There was no underground city, just the proof that people were living in the tunnels, but we had gained some precious insider's knowledge on America's, the world's poster child for the throw-away society, social mores, and eating habits. Like James, Brooklyn mainly ate food she found in dumpsters. They were both precursors of what was to become a movement in America: Freeganism. Thanks to his can collecting, James had money to buy his own food but, like freegans, he was intentionally stepping outside of mainstream consumer culture thereby reducing the grotesque wastefulness of America's hyper consumerist society. James and Brooklyn had to "dive in the dumpsters" to feed themselves but ironically, their actions had a political dimension of which they were unaware. According to researchers at the University of Arizona, the average American family discards 1.28 pounds of food a day, about 470 pounds per household per year, or 14 percent of all food brought into the house. This accounts for $43 billion in lost value. Living on the edges of society, James and Brooklyn were clear examples of the human element of America's disposable culture.

Dandelion Salad with Bacon and Potatoes
Serves 4

- Enough young dandelion leaves for 4 salads
- 4 strips of bacon
- 4 potatoes
- 1 shallot, finely chopped
- 4 eggs
- 3 tablespoons of olive oil
- 2 tablespoons of balsamic vinegar
- 1 teaspoon of Dijon mustard
- Salt and freshly ground pepper

1. Wash the dandelion leaves really well. Spin to dry and set aside.
2. Cook your potatoes in some salted water. Bring to a boil and cook until the potatoes are slightly tender.
3. Cook in a saucepan filled with water the 4 eggs until hard-boiled, remove and place them in cold water until they cool down enough to peel.
4. Cut the bacon strips into small pieces.
5. In a skillet, cook the bacon over medium heat, stirring, until crisp and brown.
6. Mix the olive oil, balsamic vinegar, mustard, finely chopped shallots with salt and black pepper together in a bowl to form a vinaigrette.
7. Peel your cooked potatoes while they are still warm and coarsely mash them with a fork.
8. Pour the dressing over the dandelion greens. Crumble the bacon on top and serve with the hot potatoes. Garnish with the chopped hard boiled eggs.

Stone soup
(With a medley of vegetables)

- 1 large well washed stone (whole)
- 3 white potatoes, peeled and chopped
- 2 sweet potatoes, peeled and chopped
- 2 carrots, peeled and chopped
- ½ head of cauliflower, chopped
- 1 handful of spinach, washed
- 2 endives, chopped
- 1 red pepper and 1 green pepper, chopped
- 1 handful of fresh kale
- 3 garlic cloves, diced
- 2 onions, chopped
- 1 celery stalk, chopped
- 4 tomatoes, diced
- Some leftover quinoa
- Some leftover black beans
- 1 pinch each of turmeric, cumin, salt and pepper
- Fresh parsley or cilantro, cut for garnish

1. Place stone inside a large cooking pot, fill with water and bring to a boil.
2. Add white and sweet potatoes, carrots, cauliflower, onions, garlic, peppers and celery.
3. Simmer for about one hour.
4. Add endives, spinach, kale, tomatoes, leftover quinoa and leftover black beans.
5. Add turmeric, cumin, salt and pepper.
6. Simmer for another fifteen minutes or so.
7. Remove from heat.
8. Remove stone and place to the side.
9. Blend in cooking pot with hand-held blender or serve as is.
10. Garnish with parsley or cilantro.
11. Serve with cheese and fresh bread to hungry villagers on a cold autumn night under the stars.

Tarte aux pommes (Apple Tart)
Serves 8

- 7 large apples (preferably organic)

Ingredients for the sweet pastry dough:

- 2½ cups of all-purpose flour
- ½ cup of sugar
- ½ cup of margarine and 1 tablespoon of margarine
- 1 egg

Making the pastry dough:

1. In a mixing bowl, mix the margarine, the sugar and the egg until creamy.
2. Add the flour. Mix the mixture with the hands altogether to form a dough into a ball.
3. Leave it to rest for an hour or two covered with a dish cloth.
4. Preheat the oven to 375°F.
5. Peel all the apples, cut in half and remove the cores.
6. In a saucepan, add a little water and cook on medium heat 3 chopped apples until soft.
7. Remove the purée from heat and set aside.
8. Brush a pie pan with margarine and roll out the dough with a rolling pin onto the pie pan.
9. Press the dough to form the pattern of the pan and arrange the apple purée over the base of the pastry shell.
10. Slice the 4 remaining apples lengthwise as thinly as possible.
11. Arrange the sliced apples on top of the apple purée.
12. Glaze the apple top with melted butter.
13. Bake for about 45–50 minutes until the apples are caramelized and crust turns golden.

Chapter Eleven

Slow and Steady Wins the Race

W e spent the next few days finishing up our article, getting it ready to send to our editor. Victorine had shot the majority of her photos in black and white and they captured the mood of my text perfectly. A strange uneasiness was nagging at me though and I discovered that Victorine felt it too.

"*Natasha, I have to get out of here,*" she said as she stood over the sink, filling the teakettle.

"*Well, call Natalie and see if she wants to meet at the coffee shop. She said she wants to hear about the rest of our underground adventure,*" I said.

"*No, no. I mean out of the city for a while. I can't relax. All I can think about is what's going on under our feet,*" she said.

"*You mean the rats?*" I said.

"*No, not the rats,*" she said with a look of disgust on her face, "*although they are a part of it. It's just that ever since we came out of that first tunnel, this city feels different to me. Above or below ground, inside or outside I feel claustrophobic and all I can see is the filth around us. Plus, let's face it. The people we've been talking to, like James and Brooklyn, have more than money issues. They had mental issues too."*

I nodded silently, thinking about her words as she paced the kitchen floor waiting for the water to boil.

"This is no way for people to live, crowded together like ants or bees in a hive . . ."

"Or rats?" I interjected.

"Exactly," she said, *"This isn't me. Papa and Mama had the right idea when they left Paris and moved to Brittany. I was trying to get out of London, now here I am living in another crowded city. I can't believe it."*

She was speaking to me but her eyes were far away. She was right. Although we both had been living in cities for the past few years, she in London and I in Paris, we were not city girls at heart. Shortly after Victorine was born, my father and mother moved out of Paris to return to his boyhood home in Brittany, the northwest of France where he, like his father, ran a small horse farm and equestrian club. That's where we grew up, in pastoral surroundings with chickens, goats, a vegetable garden, and an apple orchard in our back yard.

"Remember last week after we left the Bowery shelter, we stopped at the farmers market at Union Square on Fourteenth Street?" Victorine asked.

"Yes, of course," I said.

"Well, I was asking questions. Most of those farmers were from upstate, up near Woodstock where that famous festival was. After we submit this story let's take a drive up there and look around. I need to see some cows," she said.

Early the next Saturday morning we left New York City with no particular plan other than getting away from skyscrapers and asphalt. As we drove up the Saw Mill Parkway and found ourselves surrounded by the bright colors of the late autumn leaves, I felt a sense of calm washing over me.

"I think I had more stress in me than I realized. Let's take our time. We're not in any rush are we?" I asked.

"Okay, we'll take the back roads, maybe even find some dirt roads," answered Victorine, *"I really love this beautiful countryside. Who knows, we might find some hidden treasure."*

We drove up through the heart of the Hudson Valley, passing though historic small towns and beautiful panoramic landscapes, occasionally stopping to consult our map but mostly just avoiding highways, following our noses and turning in whatever direction seemed interesting. Along the road we found many farm stands selling fresh vegetables, eggs, and fruit. We stopped and bought a bag of apples that we munched on as we drove.

"Don't eat them all," said Victorine, *"I'm going to make an apple tart, just like Maman's when we get back."*

"Good idea," I said, remembering the treat she made from the apples from the orchard behind our house. Every fall Victorine and I would gather as many as we could, then help to peel and slice them for the naturally sweet compote Maman used for the filling. We would watch as she quickly but carefully placed the thin apple slices on top in a perfect circular pattern. When they finally came out of the oven we would wait impatiently for them to cool before gobbling them up.

"Look," I said, pointing to a road sign that read "Woodstock 12 miles," *"let's go. We can't miss that."*

Long before lending its name to the famous 1969 music festival, Woodstock was a haven for artists. In 1902, the Byrdliffe Arts Colony was established there, as a refuge from what many already thought was the dehumanizing standardization of the industrial revolution. It exists to this day as the oldest continuing arts colony in America. We spent the afternoon walking up and down Woodstock's Main Street, exploring the art galleries, boutiques, craft shops, and finally a bakery named "Bread Alone" where we found croissants that rivaled those from our favorite bakery down the street from our parent's home. We bought a half a dozen with which to indulge ourselves as we reluctantly drove home. The sun was close to setting and we were lost in thought, silently eating our croissants when we came upon a pickup truck, loaded with hay, stopped on the side of the road. Its hood was open and a man peered inside at the steaming engine. We were in a deserted area, surrounded by nothing but freshly harvested cornfields so we slowed down, stopped next to him and I rolled down my window.

"Are you in need of any help?" I asked.

A tall handsome man I judged to be in his early forties, dressed in jeans, work shirt, and baseball cap looked up from his pickup engine and smiled.

"Thanks for stopping," he said, "Seems I have a split radiator hose. Nothing I can't take care of myself but I don't have the right tools with me in the truck."

"We'll be happy to give you a lift to a service station if you would like," said Victorine.

"That's very nice of you. I really don't want to impose but what would really help me is if you could give me a lift to my farm up the road. My wife expected me about an hour ago and she's probably wondering where I am."

"Yes, of course, it's no problem," said Victorine.

"Thanks. When I get home I'll phone the local police and let them know my truck's here. Hopefully they won't ticket me," he said as he closed his hood and locked his truck. As he climbed into our back seat he said, "Hi, my name is Gary, Gary Foster."

"Hi Gary, this is Natasha and I'm Victorine, nice to meet you."

"Thanks for stopping," he said leaning forward, looking through our windshield and pointing, "So, if you turn at the next right and go straight, my farm will be up about five miles on the left. I just hope that I'm not interrupting your plans for the evening."

"Oh no, not at all, we're just taking our time driving back to the city, taking in the countryside. We're not in any hurry," I said.

"I'd just as soon not go back at all," said Victorine.

Gary didn't seem like a typical farmer. I was curious and decided to interview our new passenger.

"So Gary, what kind of farm do you have?" I asked.

"Well we have a small farm with a variety of crops but mainly we make cheese, I guess you can call us cheese artisans. We make two different kinds of cheese, 'Jersey Gold' which is a Gouda and our Blue cheese which we call 'Hudson Blues.'"

"Really? How long have you been making cheese?" said Victorine, her eyes growing wide as she smacked her lips.

"We've been making it here for about two years," he said.

"Only two years?" I asked. "Were you just farming before you started making cheese?"

"No, there's a bit of a story behind that. I should explain," he said. "This is all relatively new to us. My wife and I were, well, are, both lawyers. Three years ago we were married, living and working in New York City, at two different pretty high-profile corporate law firms. We were both doing very well financially, both on the fast track for partnership. By conventional standards we had it all, but when our daughter Grace was born, something clicked inside both of us. She was the greatest gift we were ever given . . . and a wakeup call. We wanted to bring her up in a more wholesome environment, closer to the earth . . . to be raised by us, not by a nanny. We realized we had the resources so we planned carefully and, well, at the risk of sounding trite, chose 'the road less traveled.'"

"Wow, that's a great story," I said, "Victorine and I grew up on a farm. It's wonderful place for a child."

"I think it's one of the best choices we ever made. Our friends in town thought we were crazy . . . wait, no, I take that back. Our true friends understood and support our choice but other people we knew just didn't get it. Life is very different here, we are miles away from taxis and subways and smog. We breathe clean air, are in constant symbiosis with nature. Although the homes are spread far apart, it's a close-knit community. People have each other here, along with a deeply held pride in community and family. The beauty of plain living has been largely lost in the city and even suburbia."

"Yes," said Victorine. "I totally agree."

"We don't have to worry about burglars at night, just raccoons scavenging," he said with a laugh, "We eat what we grow from the soil and know we planted the seeds. Ah, here we are now, take the next dirt driveway on your left."

Gary was quite carried away by the explanation of his new life and I must admit it was fascinating and admirable for someone to leave his career behind and start a new life with a totally new profession. Victorine turned into the dirt driveway and parked the car. In front of us stood a two-story white clapboard farmhouse with a porch that wrapped around its entire front. To the right of the house was a large red barn, as typical as you one could imagine and next to it was a little field with two white sheep covered with brown dots.

"Look at those crazy sheep," said Victorine, "I've never seen them with brown dots like that."

"Those are a couple of Jacobs' sheep that were given to us by another farmer, a friend of ours," said Gary. "Aren't they cute? They mow our lawn. Grace loves them. Come inside and let me introduce you to Sheryl and Grace."

We followed him around to the rear of the house. Standing outside the back door was a tall attractive woman with long blonde hair pulled back in a ponytail. She was wearing old jeans and an oversize men's flannel work shirt and looked to be in her late-thirties.

"Hello," she said with a puzzled look on her face.

"Honey, this is Natasha and Victorine," Gary quickly explained, "the truck broke down on route two-o-nine and they stopped to offer me a ride."

"Is it still there?" Sheryl asked excitedly, "What's wrong with it? Did you get it off of the road? When are you going to . . .?"

"It's fine, it's fine, it's off the road and it's just a radiator hose. I'll fix it in the morning," Gary answered.

Sheryl took a breath, smiled, and looked at us.

"I'm sorry. I was a bit worried. I expected my husband an hour ago. Thank you for bringing him home. Nice to meet you Natasha, nice to meet you Victoria," she said as she shook our hands.

"Nice to meet you too," said Victorine, "my name is Vic-tor-ine."

"Oh, I'm sorry, Victorine, what a lovely name, Victorine," she said, then turning to Gary, "Darling, her name is Victorine . . . not Victoria."

"Yes, I know," he said, "Where's Grace?"

"She should be up soon. She was tired out from chasing the sheep around the yard so I let her nap a bit longer."

"Would you mind waiting here for a moment?" Gary asked us, "I'll be right back."

Gary led Sheryl into the house. A few moments later they returned smiling hand in hand.

"Mademoiselles," said Gary, "I have an offer. We would like to invite you to stay for dinner and to spend the night in our guest room. It'll be dark soon and we'd hate to see you driving on these back roads at night."

"Yes, please stay," added Sheryl with a nod that looked sincere.

Victorine turned to me with a huge grin as she quickly nodded and said, "That would be very nice. We would love to stay, right Natasha?"

"Yes, we would love to, thank you," I said.

"Okay, great, why don't you come with me? I'll show you around the farm and you can help gather the food for tonight's meal."

"Honey, they're our guests," said Sheryl glaring at Gary, "You aren't going to make them work in the garden. Besides, maybe they want to freshen up after their drive."

"Oh, no. Thank you, but we're fine," said Victorine, "I want to see your farm."

"Yes, we'll be happy to help," I said, "we can do farm work. We grew up on a horse farm. This is all familiar and reminds us of home. Just tell us what you need."

Gary smiled. He seemed excited and proud to show us around.

"Okay, This is our cheese house, or our 'Chateau Fromage' as we like to call it," said Gary, chuckling to himself as he walked us towards a large white building behind the house. It looked new and didn't quite match the older house and barn.

"When we moved in, we first had to construct an industrial cheese-making facility. It took almost a year to complete with all the preparation, licensing, permits, ground testing, digging the septic, the well. Let's go inside. The facility has a lab room and three different aging rooms that operate at different temperatures and humidity levels, depending on the type of cheese. We have three eighty-gallon kettles and a one-hundred-sixty-gallon kettle to heat up the raw milk that we pump in from an outside tank. The milk is slowly heated, rennet is added, and then the mixture takes on a "Jell-O" like consistency. We use a custom-made cheese harp to slice it. The curd is then removed, placed into molds, stacked and pressed. The cheese gets flipped and brushed regularly, first with salt water and then with just a brush. The finished

Gouda wheels weigh between ten and twelve pounds. We cut the wheels and package them in slices or sell the whole wheels to restaurants."

"Wow, how did you learn to make cheese?" asked Victorine.

"Well, we just kind of got interested while we were still living and working in the city. We started reading everything we could find on the subject. Sheryl and I coordinated our vacations and time off to take cheese-making classes in Vermont. We started making small batches in our apartment and even went to France for a cheese tour. Our friends teased us but we just loved it too much to care. We looked at each other one day and we both just knew we were ready to do this full time. After having learned about various varieties we chose to manufacture raw milk cheese, which has to age for sixty days."

I watched Victorine as she listened to Gary and noticed an odd expression on her face.

"We make our cheese very much in the European tradition," said Gary, "I'm sure you know, nothing much is pasteurized there unless it's on an industrial scale. We hand craft cheese that's made from fresh, hormone-free cow's milk which we get it from two different local farms."

"Where do you market your cheese?" I asked.

"Well, this year we're at three weekly farmers markets and we're also trying to market to local wineries. We have a few restaurants that buy from us but our operation remains small at the moment."

"It's not easy to make cheese, but it's certainly easy to eat it," said Victorine, "I am hoping that you'll get my hint and let us try some."

"Yes, you can say that it's not easy but we love doing it and of course, I was hoping you'll sample some and give us your honest opinion. With a French palate, I'm sure you know your cheeses ... Oh look, my little girl's awake. Come give Daddy a kiss, come on my Gracie."

Sheryl walked in carrying an adorable little girl with golden locks who was wiping sleep from her eyes with chubby little fists. Sheryl placed her gently on the ground and she toddled on unsteady legs over to Gary while Sheryl followed close behind.

"Yes, Miss Gracie is still waking up," Sheryl said, "Look Sweetie, we have two guests today from far away. This is Natasha and Victorine."

"Hello Gracie," we sang in unison as we crouched down and smiled.

Gracie giggled, grabbed her father's leg and hid her face in the fabric of his jeans.

"She's adorable," I said.

"Yes, she's my sunshine," said Sheryl, "Gracie and I are going back to the kitchen to get dinner started."

"Ok Honey, we'll be in soon with the vegetables," said Gary, giving both Gracie and Sheryl a kiss on the cheek.

Sheryl picked up Gracie and left while Gary continued with his tour outside in the garden.

"Cheese isn't the only product we sell from the farm. We have the eggs from two dozen chickens which we sell at farmers markets and Sheryl cans peppers, tomatoes, green beans, and pickles, and makes salsa and pesto made from our own fresh Genoa basil. We grow our vegetables on the two acres of land over there," he said pointing out behind the barn.

"Canning is Sheryl's department," continued Gary, "She does quite well at it and it keeps her busy. We can our winter reserve as much as possible and this winter we expect to feed ourselves almost totally from our own garden. We're proud locavores, try to eat in season and as fresh as we can. Right through our final harvest we pick vegetables from our garden for each meal. Our meat comes from a local farmer who raises grass-fed cattle and the poultry comes from another local farm where they raise free-range chickens. We also barter as much as possible."

"This is how everybody should eat and live. Return to the land and the old ways just like our grandparents did," I said.

"Have you heard of the slow food movement?" Gary asked.

"The slow food movement?" I repeated.

"Yes, I've heard about it," said Victorine. "I know it started in Italy but I can't remember the name of the man who started the movement."

"Yes, yes, that's right," said Gary, "it was founded in Italy by Carlo Petrini in 1986 as a way to oppose fast food and to promote the heritage, traditions, and culture of food."

"Yes I know. My goal was . . . is to live that way," said Victorine sighing, "It's about buying local, raising food in a sustainable way free of synthetic chemicals, fertilizers and pesticides and farm animals are raised in a humane way outdoors."

Sheryl called Gary from the kitchen window, "I am about ready, I need those vegetables. Why don't you come get Gracie and take Natasha and Victorine to pick some collard greens and spinach, oh, and bring me some arugula and basil."

Sheryl disappeared from the window then quickly returned adding, "please."

"Okay Honey," Gary called to Sheryl, and then to us, "I'll be right back."

Gary trotted up to the house and disappeared in the back door.

"I'm so glad his truck broke down," I said, *"The last thing I wanted to do tonight was go back to our apartment."*

"Yes, they seem nice," said Victorine, *"I wonder how much they had to put into this place. They must have had some start-up money."*

"They were both Manhattan lawyers," I said, *"I'm sure they planned this very well and have a nice reserve put away."*

Gary returned carrying Gracie and two wicker baskets. He handed me one basket and handed Gracie to Victorine who carried her around on her hip as we walked through the rows of vegetables harvesting our dinner. As the light faded with the setting sun Gary quickly filled our baskets.

"One of my greatest pleasures now is walking in this garden and seeing the fruits of our labors growing here at our feet," said Gary, surveying the rows of vegetables. "It may sound corny but honestly, one harvest is more rewarding than all the years I spent working in the city."

As I listened to Gary, my thoughts drifted to memories of our countless childhood visits to my grandmother's garden. Victorine and I would lift the net covering her miniature strawberry field and steal as many strawberries as we could carry. Our grandmother was a grocer who sold her garden's fruits and vegetables at the weekly town market. I fondly remembered their apple orchard where we would sit under the trees and eat the most delicious apples. With these recollections, I felt a pang of guilt. What had happened to us in America? We were eating unconsciously, without thought. Stopping for takeout burgers and eating them while driving had become de rigueur, something we would never, ever think of doing back at home. We had drifted away from sitting down to regular meals and instead taken up the habit of "grazing" throughout the day. The microwave had become the most used appliance in our kitchen. The act of eating had become mindless and I felt an odd stirring deep inside as we approached the kitchen with our mini harvest.

"Oh good, perfect timing," said Sheryl as we entered the back door, "I started a potato salad. Victorine, could you finish it for me? Just wash and mince up some basil and dill and add it with olive oil, balsamic vinegar, a little salt and pepper. I'm going to sauté some collard greens with shallots and garlic. Natasha, could you wash the spinach and the arugula for the salad? We'll crumble in some Blue cheese, that should be tasty, oh, and could you slice up and add some onions too."

Sheryl handed Gracie to Gary and with two hands free she worked fast. While the collard greens simmered, she cracked and whisked a half dozen eggs in a bowl, diced some mushrooms and onions, browned them in a sauce pan, added the beaten eggs with herbs, and came up with a delicious-looking omelet. The aroma of the food began to make my mouth water. Victorine was unusually quiet, deep in thought and just not acting her typical self.

I watch Gary and Gracie as they set the large kitchen table. As he lay down each plate and bowl, they counted together.

"One," said Gary.

"Un," repeated Gracie.

"Two."

"Doo."

"Three."

"Tree . . ."

It was slow going with the counting lesson but they finished just as Sheryl announced dinner was ready. We sat down to our meal: potato salad, collard greens, arugula and spinach salad with blue cheese and heirloom tomatoes, and a tomato-mushroom-herb omelet.

"Bon appétit," I said, reaching for a slice of bread.

"Sheryl baked the bread this morning," said Gary as he passed me a plate of cheese, "and please try some of our homemade Gouda."

"Mmm, this is delicious, it really is. It tastes just like home, Victorine. Try it," I said, snatching a second slice before passing her the plate.

"There's homemade lemonade and iced tea in the fridge if you like. Please just help yourself," said Sheryl who had her hands full feeding and balancing Gracie on her lap.

The smells and tastes of the freshly baked bread and garden vegetables on the table were delicious. I took another bite of the homemade cheese and felt like Proust biting into his now famous madeleine. It brought back memories of my mother's kitchen. She would have been shocked if she knew the horrible way we had been eating the last few months.

"I must say that it's been a long time since we've sat down to a proper meal like this. We've kind of lost our way with food here in America," I said looking at Victorine sheepishly.

She nodded slightly without looking up.

"I can understand that. I fell into the same sort of situation," said Sheryl, "For me it was the first time I left home for college when I was eighteen. I felt very scared, lost and alone and began eating compulsively. It wasn't just the typical 'freshman fifteen' as they say. I really lost touch with my natural intuition and ignored what my body was telling me. When I gained weight I started to feel guilty and food became an enemy. It was a vicious circle but I finally got help when I realized food wasn't the root of my problem. There were some other deeper issues that had to be addressed."

"That's what's happening to me," Victorine said softly.

"That's what happened to a lot of people in this country," Sheryl said, "It's become a cliché but it's true, you are what you eat. That's one of the reasons we moved out here, to be close to the earth. Awareness of where your food comes from is one cornerstone of a healthy attitude towards eating. We want Gracie to know that vegetables grow from the ground and that milk comes from a cow, not from the cartons in the store."

"Moo, moo," Gracie suddenly sang out.

Gary reached over and lifted Gracie from Sheryl's lap and placed her in his own.

"That's right my little lamb, and what do the sheep say?" he asked.

"Bah, bah," she answered before bursting into giggles.

To my surprise, Gracie was eating the same food as we adults, a bit of collard greens, a bit of omelet and even some blue cheese.

"It's amazing for Gracie to like a strong cheese like that," I said as Gracie devoured her third helping of blue cheese and licked her fingers.

"Yes, we have strong beliefs on this subject," said Sheryl. "That's why from an early age, well, since she was an infant, we've consistently fed her whole foods. When I started breast-feeding I was extra careful about my own diet. I did a lot of research while pregnant and learned that some doctors believe doing so metabolically programs children on a cellular level to make healthy food choices later on in life. They say that after two or three years of a diet like this, children will naturally be able to distinguish healthy choices from bad based on how their body feels. They themselves will recognize differences in things ranging from digestion to emotions and social interactions."

Victorine suddenly jumped up from the table and ran out of the kitchen. I heard the bathroom door close in the hall then a muffled sobbing. Gary, Sheryl, and I sat frozen for a moment, looking at each other wide eyed. Gary asked very softly, "Is she okay?"

I listened again and heard what water running and splashing in the sink.

"Yes, I think she's okay, Let's give her a few minutes," I whispered, "We've had an emotional few weeks. I think this trip today has dredged up some memories for both of us."

"I understand," Sheryl whispered, then to Gary, "Honey, why don't you take Gracie up for her bath."

Gary nodded but before he could move I heard the bathroom door open and Victorine walked back into the kitchen and returned to her seat at the table. Her eyes were red and puffy but she had composed herself.

"I'm sorry," she said softly, "I lost it for a moment. Please, don't mind me."

Gracie stared at Victorine curiously. We watched silently as she wriggled down off her father's lap and made her way slowly around the table till she was standing directly next to Victorine. Victorine smiled softly and looked at her through misty eyes as Gracie reached up, took Victorine's hand and gently stroked it. Victorine scooped up Gracie in her arms and buried her face in her blonde curls. No one spoke as Gary and I cleared the table and Sheryl filled the teakettle and placed it on the burner. She then touched Gary's arm, gave him a look, and motioned with her head toward Victorine and Gracie. He gently lifted Gracie from Victorine's lap and said, "Okay kiddo, it's time for your bath."

They left the kitchen and I heard his footsteps ascend the stairs and fade away.

"*What's wrong? Are you okay?*" I asked as Sheryl turned and began preparing a pot of tea.

"*Yes, I'm fine but don't speak French, it's not polite,*" she answered.

"Shall I leave you two alone so you can talk?" asked Sheryl.

"No, no, no, please don't go," said Victorine as her eyes began tearing up again, "I'm so sorry for ruining your lovely dinner. You must think I'm crazy."

She sat in her chair looking totally deflated. Sheryl set a tray with three mugs, a honey jar, and a large teapot down on the table. She then sat down next to Victorine.

"Don't be silly. Listen, I'm going to let you in on a little secret," she said leaning a little closer and lowering her voice, "you're not the first woman who's suddenly burst into tears for no apparent reason."

Victorine laughed through her tears and wiped her eyes with her napkin as the kettle began to whistle on the stove. Sheryl got up, turned off the flame, returned with the kettle, and filled the teapot.

"Seriously, have some tea and if you want to talk, I'm all ears," Sheryl said as she covered the steeping teapot with a cozy.

Victorine looked at us both then took a breath and let out a long sigh.

"I don't know," she began, "I was so happy when I first saw your farm, then, when we started preparing dinner something came over me and I became, well, unbelievably sad watching the two of you with Gracie. It's just that, well, this, this life is what we . . . what I planned, the life I thought we would . . ."

Tears welled up in Victorine's eyes and she sat with her head lowered, sobbing softly. Sheryl looked across the table at me and raised her eyebrows. She didn't say a word and I stayed silent also. She poured a mug of tea, stirred some honey into it and placed it in front of Victorine. Sheryl poured a tea for me and herself as Victorine composed herself. It dawned on me that she was talking about Nigel, a subject that had previously been off limits. All I had heard about their break-up was what our mother had related to me. Anytime I brought it up Victorine just changed subjects. Now the story was coming out diluted with tears.

" . . . the life I imagined we would be living," continued Victorine, "I'm sorry, I'm not making sense."

"No, that's fine, take your time," said Sheryl, sliding Victorine's mug closer.

Victorine took a sip of tea then a deep breath and relaxed into her chair.

"Before Natasha and I came to America, I was living in London with . . ." Victorine hesitated then continued after a long sigh, "I was living in London with my boyfriend, Nigel. We met when I was at university studying ecological science. I fell for him quickly and before I knew what had happened we moved into a flat together. With help from one of his old school chums we managed to obtain a lease hold on a row house in the North End. Financially it made sense to buy rather than rent, but I always considered it temporary. I never had any intention of living in London my whole life. Nigel's family had a small non-working farm, about two or two and a half hours west of London in Wiltshire, near a village named Bradford on Avon. It was beautiful. We would drive out there to visit whenever we could. We made plans to move there when I finished my degree. We talked about creating a little farm much like you have here . . . getting back to living close to the land . . . I planned an herb garden . . . a hen house . . ."

Victorine's voice trailed off. She had stopped crying and her eyes were now fixed on a distant place in front of her, lost in a memory. She jolted herself out of her thoughts, took a sip of tea, and continued her story.

"Nigel's a musician. He played in pubs. He wasn't earning much so I bought a little van and we started a dog-walking service together. My idea was to tuck the money we earned from that away into a little farm fund. I worked hard, so ... so ... hard ... to save as much money as possible. We seldom ate out or spent money on anything except necessities."

Victorine was now becoming more animated. I realized that the words now pouring out of her were a synopsis of the pent-up frustration and anger that had been swirling around inside her head ever since we left France.

"When I finally I got my diploma I began taking steps to put the plan in motion," she continued, "I took another job in the evenings to cover our daily expenses and told Nigel I wanted to put the house on the market. He said we should wait, not rush into it. That's when I should have woken up ... but I didn't. Then, without telling me he used some of our savings to bring his band into the recording studio ... then he bought a new guitar ... that's when I REALLY should have woken up ... but still I didn't. We started to fight about the money. He would say, 'but Luv, a big booking agent's coming tonight. If he likes the band we'll have a record deal and won't have to think about money.' It happened over and over and over and I just let it. They say love is blind but for me it was also deaf and dumb. I made myself believe he wanted the same thing I did ... then ... I finally woke up. Living in London and having a country place a few hours away to go to once in a while was enough for him. He had no intention of moving to a farm or even leaving London ... it was my dream, not his."

Victorine let out a long sigh and stared into her mug. I sat silent, digesting the information I had just heard. I couldn't wait to be alone with a telephone so I could call our mother. Sheryl took a deep breath and cleared her throat.

"Well, that's a difficult realization to reach but I think it was very healthy. Still, it doesn't make it any less painful," she said, "Is he out of the picture now?"

"Yes." answered Victorine, "When it hit me, I sort of left the relationship without actually leaving ... I just checked out. We lived together but we were basically roommates. He finally cheated on me. It gave me an excuse to officially end it . . . I almost have to thank him for that. He even offered to leave and let me stay in the house but I said no. I just wanted to be out of there, out of London, out of . . . anything I knew. I wanted to get as far away as possible. That's the real reason I came here to America . . .”

Victorine turned her head and looked at me for the first time since she began her story.

“ . . . Yes, that's the real reason . . . and I dragged Natasha along with me.”

She gave a little shrug and a smile. I just smiled back. Upstairs I heard doors opening and closing and footsteps, big and small.

“Well,” said Sheryl, “It sounds like Miss Gracie has finished her bath. How would you two like to help me get her to bed?”

“I'd like nothing more,” said Victorine as I nodded eagerly.

That night, in Gary and Sheryl's guest bedroom, Victorine snored softly next to me as I lay awake thinking about our day and my future. Maybe I had been dragged along to America but I was glad of it. Thanks to Victorine I had also been given a new start . . . a new start and a chance to gain back my confidence. I was proud of the mole people story we had just submitted but I was now ready to move on. Over the past months I had been making inquiries and had scheduled an appointment the following week. I was thinking about my upcoming interview at the United Nations.

Mushroom Omelette
Serves 4

- 8 large eggs, preferably organic or free-range
- 8 to 10 mushrooms of your choice
- 2 tablespoons of unsalted butter
- 2 shallots
- 1 sprig of parsley
- sea salt and freshly ground pepper

1. Crack the eggs into a mixing bowl.
2. Add a pinch of salt and pepper.
3. Beat well with a fork.
4. Chop the mushrooms and add to a large frying pan on a high heat with some of the butter.
5. Fry and toss around until golden, then turn the heat down to medium.
6. Add the eggs and move the pan around to spread them out evenly.
7. Beat the eggs thoroughly along with the salt and fresh ground pepper.
8. Chop the shallots finely.
9. Heat a little of the butter in a pan and toss the shallots until golden then add the washed and sliced mushrooms.
10. Remove the mushrooms and keep aside.
11. Melt the remaining butter in a non-stick pan over a medium flame and add the beaten eggs to it.
12. Spread evenly around the pan and sprinkle the mushrooms on top.
13. When it starts to turn golden brown underneath, remove the pan from the heat and slide the omelet onto a plate.

Goat Cheese Cake
Serves 12

- 6 oz. of unbleached, all purpose flour
- 3 large eggs
- 2 tablespoons of olive oil
- 2 teaspoons of baking yeast
- 4 oz. of grated comté cheese
- 3 chèvre cheese crottins (approx. 12 oz.)
- 1 cup of whole milk (warm)
- 3 oz. of shelled walnut
- 2 oz. of raisins
- Pinch of sea salt and fresh pepper

1. Put the raisins in lukewarm water for fifteen minutes until they plump up.
2. Beat the chèvre in a large bowl until smooth and mixed well, set aside.
3. In another bowl beat the eggs, flour, yeast, salt and pepper.
4. Slowly add the olive oil and the warm whole milk mixing well.
5. Add the grated cheese and beat well.
6. Add the chèvre and crushed walnuts.
7. Drain water from and the raisins and add to batter and mix well.
8. Pour the batter evenly in a rectangular buttered cake mold.
9. Bake approximately 40 minutes or until the outer edge of the cake is puffed.
10. Remove the cake from the oven and let it cool for 15 minutes.

Soupe aux Orties (Wild nettles soup)
Serves 6

- 8 cups of water
- 1 pound nettles, washed, leaves picked
- 1 pound potatoes, peeled and chopped
- 1 large onion, chopped
- 4 garlic cloves, diced
- 3 tablespoons of butter
- ½ cup of crème fraîche or sour cream
- 1 tablespoon of salt
- 1 tablespoon of freshly ground pepper
- ¼ tablespoon of curcuma

1. Wearing rubber gloves, prepare the nettles, trim the stems out of the nettles you have picked, leaving just the fresh, young leaves. Wash and drain them.
2. Melt the butter in a large saucepan over medium heat. Add the onion, garlic and cook for 5 minutes, stirring occasionally until the onion and garlic are soft.
3. Add potatoes and the water and simmer for a further 20 minutes.
4. Add the nettles and cook for another 10 minutes.
5. Remove from the heat. Puree the soup using an electric hand-held blender. Season to taste, then stir in some of the crème fraîche.
6. To serve, pour the soup into a bowl and add some cream with some curcuma. Swirl the cream with the curcuma around with the back of a spoon to make an interesting shape.

Tip: Wear gloves to save yourself from getting stung when foraging for wild nettles. They grow in abundance and are best eaten in the spring before they flower. The taste of nettle soup varies considerably depending on the "terroir" of the nettles, how warm the weather is, and what stage of growth of the plant.

Chapter Twelve

The Quickest Way
to the Heart . . .

I t was around dusk and I was sitting at our little kitchen table with a cup of tea, editing my résumé when Victorine, bundled up in her hat, scarf, and mittens, burst through the front door.

"I've made a complete fool of myself today, you have no idea . . ." she said as she plopped her grocery bag on the kitchen table and disappeared into the bedroom.

"So, another typical day, huh?" I called after her.

She didn't hear me or was simply ignoring me and returned wearing her house slippers and comfy robe.

" . . . Let me tell you. You'll get a good kick out of this, Ouf, I'm still flustered . . ." she continued as she unpacked her bag and carefully placed each item on the table.

"But let me tell you, that's it, that's IT. I've started my new protocol. I'm back to my old ways, no more meat or junk food . . ."

I reached to examine one of the containers.

"Just wait, just wait and listen," she said, smacking my hand away and sliding the containers out of my reach.

Victorine wanted my full attention so I crossed my arms, leaned back in my chair and listened to her story.

"As you know, I've turned into a carnivore these last weeks, or rather last months and the consequences have been tragic. Well, I stopped at the market on the way home and without even thinking, picked up a whole roast chicken. I paid at the register but as I was leaving the store I saw a reflection in the window. I thought, wow, look at that fat cow, but then, I realized it was me! Natasha, I didn't even recognize myself. It suddenly hit me . . . I have to change my diet and should definitely not be eating a single piece of meat anymore, so, I went back inside and told the cashier I wanted to return my chicken. That shouldn't be so difficult, right?"

"Yeah, go on," I said, wondering where this was going.

"She said, 'well I don't know . . . I have to call my manager.'"

Victorine's impersonation of the cashier was spot on. I knew exactly which girl she was talking about and we both laughed before she continued.

"So, she waited for the manager to come and void the purchase. He took forever and the people in line behind me were becoming impatient. Some of them began complaining out loud. The idiots were grumbling and say-ing 'come on, let's go, let's go.' I was already upset and getting more and more flustered. The guy right behind me must have noticed it because he very calmly whispered, 'don't worry about those jerks, there's no rush.'"

Victorine's story was getting interesting and she now had my full attention.

"He then asked me, 'What's wrong with the chicken?' I told him just what I told you, that I decided at that very moment to go back to being a vegetarian. He then asked, 'then what are you going to do for dinner' and I said, 'I don't know yet, but I WON'T be eating chicken.' The manager finally arrived, punched in his special refund code and the cashier returned my money. I started to leave when the calm guy said, 'wait a second, let me check out and I'll tell you about a great place to get some takeout vegetarian food.' He paid for his bunch of bananas and bottle of water, put them in his backpack, and

followed me outside. He told me there was a great new vegetarian place just one block out of his way. He offered to walk me over there on his way to the subway. He was right. It's called Suzi's Kitchen. *Look what I got . . ."*

Victorine ceremoniously opened her takeout containers one by one.

"*. . . vegetarian Vietnamese summer rolls. Remember? Just like we used to get in Paris . . . seaweed and kale salad with silken tofu and ginger vinaigrette dressing, and taste this soup, just what my body has been craving for so long."*

I took the spoon from my mug and tasted the soup. It was good, a simple miso base with thick noodles and lots of scallions.

"*Why didn't you just go to Sami's and get a hummus and tabouleh salad?*" I asked, reaching for a second helping of soup.

"*I told you I'm never going back to that place,*" she answered, pointing at me with her fork, "*Besides, this is so much better.*"

Sadly, after our fiasco at Sami's, we had neglected to explore all the great restaurants in New York, a multicultural city where you can find anything your palate desires. Over the next few weeks, while Victorine got herself back on her vegetarian regimen, we splurged and became regulars at Suzi's. As for me, I resolved to eat only organic meat and vegetables and cut out junk food. We both resolved to stop eating on the run and sit down to all our meals. We went on an expedition and found all the greengrocers in a three-block radius of our apartment. Finally, we unplugged our microwave and vowed to let it collect dust. Then, one afternoon a few weeks later, as we sat eating lunch at Suzi's, Victorine froze in mid-sentence with her mouth open and her tofu-laden fork suspended in the air as she stared over my shoulder at the entrance.

"*There he is Natasha, there, that's him,*" she whispered excitedly.

"*Who, who are you talking about?*" I asked.

"*The guy from the market, who brought me here the first time,*" she whispered, "*he's at the entrance right now.*"

I turned to look and saw standing at the entrance an attractive man with a large musical instrument case slung over his shoulder. He smiled when he spotted Victorine and walked straight over to our table.

"See, I told you you'd come back," he said.

Victorine, uncharacteristically at a loss for words just nodded, "uh-huh."

They stared at each for a long moment and I began to wonder if I was invisible.

"Aren't you going to introduce us?" I asked Victorine.

"Oh, I'm sorry, my name's Jude," he said, "I didn't mean to interrupt your lunch."

"No, no, not at all, I'm Natasha . . ." I said extending my hand, " . . . and I understand you've already met Victorine. She told me you recommended this restaurant. Thank you, it's wonderful, we've come here almost every day this week."

"Yes, thank you," said Victorine, finally finding her voice, "I was in a dreadful state that evening and you directed me to just the right place. This seaweed and kale salad has become my favorite item on the menu. It's like medicine for me."

"Good, I'm glad I could help," said Jude, "Now, let me guess. Sisters?"

We nodded in unison. I looked over and noticed a sparkle in Victorine's eyes that had been absent for a long time. It could understand her being tongue-tied. Jude was very handsome with chin-length dark hair, huge expressive green eyes, and a relaxed manner. Now that he was closer I could see that he was carrying a cello case over his shoulder.

"Would you like to join us?" I said, motioning to our table's empty chair.

"Oh, thank you, I'd really like to," he said, "but I'm just stopping in to grab something to go. I'm on my way to rehearsal for a performance tonight. Maybe we could meet later this evening . . . or . . . I have an idea . . ."

His face lit up as reached into a side pocket of his cello case, pulled out a postcard and handed it to Victorine.

" . . . if you're both free tonight you might like to come to my show. I'm playing at Joe's Pub with an American singer who lived in Paris for ten years and now does a tribute to Edith Piaf. She's not bad. I could put you on the guest list . . ."

He paused for a moment as Victorine examined the postcard.

"Tell you what. I'll go order my food while you decide. I'll be back and you can let me know."

Over Victorine's shoulder I watched Jude order at the counter then step to the rear, pull out his cell phone, and make a call.

Victorine handed me the postcard and nodded.

"Yes Natasha, let's go. It sounds like fun," she whispered.

I had some reading and translation exercises I had planned to do that evening to prepare for my upcoming interview at the United Nations, but I decided to let it wait. I wanted to see if that sparkle in Victorine's eyes would get any brighter.

"Okay," I said, *"let's go."*

Jude returned to our table with his takeout bag.

"Well, what's the verdict?" asked Jude.

"Yes, we would love to come," said Victorine.

"Good, I'm glad," he said, with a little chuckle, "I took a chance, called and reserved the tickets. So, the show is at nine thirty at Joe's Pub, the address is on the card I gave you. Two tickets will be waiting for you at the box office under my name, Jude Elder. I hope you enjoy it. If you wait for me afterward we can go grab a drink or a bite to eat if you like. We can pick up where we left off. I'd like to hear how two French sisters wound up here in Astoria, Queens."

Jude said goodbye and promptly left with a wave and a lingering look at Victorine. Her eyes followed him out the door.

"He's interesting, not a typical American," she said, her eyes still outside.

"Yes, he's quite smooth. He just asked you out on a date without you realizing it," I said.

"Oh really? What makes you think I didn't realize it?" she asked with a sly smile.

At about eight p.m. we emerged from the subway station at Astor Place in lower Manhattan. The neighborhood, called NoHo, short for North of Houston, borders the East Village, long considered the epicenter of urban counterculture. For decades it has been a magnet for artists, musicians, writers, actors, and other free thinkers from around the world. Home to New York University, the Cooper Union School of Architecture, and countless little cafes, clubs, and art galleries, its streets are perpetually teeming with young people, alive with energy. Victorine looked at her watch.

"We have an hour before we have to pick up our tickets," she said, *"let's take a walk and check out the neighborhood."*

We strolled up and down the crowded sidewalk on St. Mark's Place, past vintage clothes stores, used book shops, coffee houses, and to our surprise a number of vegetarian restaurants. Couples arm in arm and groups of students were talking and laughing as they hurried past us. Snatches of live music could be heard emanating from clubs and restaurants as we passed.

"It's nice here. Why didn't we ever come down to this neighborhood?" asked Victorine as she leaned in to read the menu on window of a little Middle Eastern café.

"We did," I answered, *"well, close by anyway. The Bowery Mission is a few blocks away, but we were only looking for desperate homeless people then, not vegetarian food."*

Victorine looked around at the scene on the bustling street, took a deep breath, and exhaled a cloud of mist into the chilly evening air.

"You know, Papa always said, 'Be careful what you look for, because you may find it' . . ."

"Yes," I said, *"meaning?"*

She didn't answer. She just looked up towards the rooftops with a serene smile, linked arms with me and said, *"Come on, let's go pick up our tickets."*

When we entered Joe's Pub, I was immediately glad we had gone back to our apartment and changed into something a bit more elegant for the evening. Joe's Pub was not a "pub" at all but actually a sophisticated supper club with soft lighting, long banquet seats covered with red velvet cushions, and candlelit cabaret tables clustered in front of a small stage. It was named after Joseph Papp, founder of the adjoining New York Public Theater, and created as an intimate showcase venue for up and coming as well as established artists.

"Yes, two for Jude Elder, right this way," said the tall blonde hostess dressed from head to toe in black.

We followed her as she slinked her way through the maze of tables, leading us to our seats in directly in front of the stage.

"*Well, this is nice,*" I said when she left, "*I wasn't expecting it to be this elegant.*"

"*Shh, be careful what you say,*" whispered Victorine, "*listen.*"

I looked around, wondering what she was referring to. I cocked my head to listen and immediately heard it. Mixed in the murmuring of the crowd I heard snatches of conversation in French. I realized suddenly that we were at a tribute to Edith Piaf so of course the audience would be full of people who spoke French. Victorine and I had become accustomed to commenting on and critiquing our surroundings and the people in it, while we were in America, confident we couldn't be understood by those around us. We didn't have that luxury here. I kept silent and surveyed the room. On stage was a microphone on a tall stand, two empty chairs, a drum set, an upright bass lying on its side, and a black baby grand piano. I caught a few more snatches of French conversation, studied other members of the audience, and thought about what had drawn them to see this show. Arguably France's most famous singer, Edith Piaf can best be compared to American torch singers Judy Garland and Billie Holiday. She sang songs of bittersweet, doomed love . . . love that burned so fiercely it was destined to consume itself. Her interpretations of these songs are believed to be fueled by the tragedies of her own life. To this day she holds a special place in the hearts of the French, both young and old, perhaps because we carry a secret longing to experience love with the same intensity she expressed with her voice . . . a love maybe tragic, but definitely true. Since her death, a number of singers have been hailed as the "New Piaf" and have attempted to capture her unique style of interpreting a lyric. Some have even recorded her signature songs but she is still the standard to which all French female popular singers are compared.

A tall, thin, red-headed waitress with alabaster skin and bright red lipstick appeared at our table holding a tray.

"Hi, how are you tonight?" she asked, "You're Jude's guests?"

We looked at her and nodded in unison.

"There's a two-drink minimum," she said, then discreetly handing us an envelope she added with a wink and a smile, "he's left these drink tickets for you."

I ordered red wine and Victorine a pot of hot tea.

"Come on, I'm going to find the bathroom," whispered Victorine.

I glanced at my watch. It was 9:20 p.m. With our coats reserving our places on the back of our chairs, we found the ladies room and returned just as the house lights began to dim. The stage went dark but I could faintly make out shadows on it moving about, finding their places. There was a moment of stillness then the piano struck a few introductory chords. A spot light flicked on and in the narrow beam of light stood a woman with short black hair, heavy pancake makeup and deep red lipstick. She wore a simple knee-length black dress with long sleeves. The audience burst into applause and as it died away she began to sing . . .

"I live at the corner of old Montmartre

My father returns home drunk every night . . ."

I heard little gasps in the darkness around me and the audience burst into brief applause as it recognized the familiar song *"On My Street,"* about a young girl who hears the frightening sounds of prostitutes walking outside her window at night and is told by her father that one day soon she'll have to join them.

One after another she sang the classic songs made famous by the singer known as France's "Little Sparrow": "Life in Rosy Hues," "My Lord," "Hymn of Love," "It's Love," "Waltz of Love." Jude was right. She wasn't bad. No, she wasn't Piaf but it's difficult for we French to ignore the tug on our hearts when we hear anyone singing one of her iconic songs. However, what I found most entertaining was peeking over and watching Victorine. There were four other musicians onstage besides the singer but Victorine's eyes remained glued to Jude playing his cello. I could understand why. Clearly he was an accomplished musician. He played beautifully and made it look effortless but I could tell what really mesmerized her was his relaxed poise onstage. He looked like someone who had found his passion, someone who had truly learned to live in the moment. When the show ended and the ensemble tried to leave the stage, the audience wouldn't stop applauding, demanding an encore. The singer obliged with one of my favorites, "Padam, Padam", a song about the memories of lost loves that haunt us in the night. Both Victorine and I found ourselves joining in with the rest of the audience, singing the refrain. The lights came up, we left a generous tip for our waitress, collected our coats, and waited by the bar for Jude. A few minutes later he emerged from backstage.

"I'm glad you could make it," he shouted over the din of the bar crowd and music now blasting over the loudspeakers.

"Oh no, thank you," we both said, almost shouting to be heard.

"This place always turns into a just another loud bar scene after the show. Would you like to go someplace quieter? Maybe someplace where we can get a tea or coffee and actually talk?" he asked, "I know a place close by."

Victorine and I both nodded eagerly. I was curious about this unusual American and wanted to ask him a few questions. Obviously, Victorine did too. Jude slung his cello case over his shoulder, waved goodbye to his bandmates and we stepped outside. The chilly night air combined with the relative quiet of the street was refreshing. A few people who I recognized from the audience were milling about outside, chatting and smoking. They smiled and nodded at Jude as we passed. One said, "thank you," another said, "yes, beautiful playing." As we strolled down the sidewalk three abreast we thanked him again for inviting us, told him how much we enjoyed the show, how nostalgic it made us feel, and that it was just what we needed to see tonight.

"Good, I'm glad you liked it. Of course, no one can compare to Edith Piaf but Caroline's a good singer and her love of the songs really comes across . . . Ah, here it is." he said stopping in front of a dimly lit storefront a few blocks down the street. The sign above the door read "AUNT SADIE'S ATTIC."

"I like this place. It's unusual, quiet, very relaxed and . . . it's open late," said Jude.

He was right. The interior, filled with mismatched tables and chairs, bookshelf-lined walls, and an odd assortment of floor and table lamps providing soft lighting was very cozy. About a half a dozen customers were scattered around, some reading, some talking quietly. Soft jazz played in the background. An espresso machine sat on the counter in the back and the shelves behind it were filled with about two-dozen assorted vintage teapots.

"This looks more like a secondhand furniture shop than a coffee shop," I said.

"It's both," said Jude nodding with a grin, "Look closely. Everything has a price tag. The décor is always changing as things get sold then replaced with new stuff."

I looked around and now that he pointed it out, saw little white tags on all the furniture then noticed a sign on the bookshelf, "ALL PAPERBACKS-$1/ ALL HARDCOVERS-$3."

We seated ourselves in a cluster of comfy overstuffed chairs by the window while Jude tucked his cello in the corner then went to the counter to put in our order. He returned with a cappuccino for himself and a pot of tea for us.

"A cappuccino now? " asked Victorine, "how will you get to sleep?"

"Oh, I'm not going to be sleeping for a while," said Jude checking his watch, "It's only eleven o'clock. I have a recording session later."

"Later?" asked Victorine sitting up straight, "How much later?"

"Oh, I should get there a little after midnight," he said, "My friend owns a recording studio near Astor Place, close to where we just were. He also plays drums in a show on Broadway. He finished up his show a little while ago so by the time he packs up, stops for something to eat and gets home it will be about midnight. I'll head over there then."

"Wow, do you normally start working that late?" she asked.

"No, not normally but he got this last-minute session to redo the music for a TV commercial and the deadline is tomorrow . . . but wait," he said waving his hand and interrupting himself, "I don't want to talk about him. You saw and hear what I do. Now it's your turn. I want to get the story on you two. What are you doing here in New York? How long have you been here?"

He looked back and forth at both of us then his eyes came to rest on Victorine. She looked at me then back to Jude, took a deep breath, and proceeded to give him a concise yet colorful account of our adventures over the past months. I interjected a comment here and there but mostly just listened to her tell our story. She didn't embellish or exaggerate a thing. She gave an accurate description of our travels and adventures, and as Jude sat there listening his eyes grew wider and wider. When he finished he looked at both of us, shook his head, laughed and said, "That's it. You two are insane. I'm calling Bellevue and having you both committed. The KKK? Snakes? Subway tunnels? You're both lucky you're not dead."

We laughed, talked a little while longer, he asked questions, we asked questions and then he glanced at his watch and sighed.

"I'm sorry, really I have to get going but I'd love to see your photographs Victorine. Can I call you?" he asked.

We exchanged phone numbers then he walked us to our subway station and bid us both good night with a kiss on both cheeks in the typical European fashion. He waved and disappeared into the crowd of the still bustling Astor Place.

"*I like him. I'd like to see him again,*" said Victorine.

"*Don't worry. You will,*" I said, grabbing her arm and leading her down the stairs to the subway platform.

Late afternoon the next day, Saturday, I was sitting at our kitchen table reading and going over some translation exercises when the phone rang. Victorine picked it up in the bedroom and I heard her muffled voice behind the door. A few minutes later she came out and stood in the kitchen doorway.

"*Guess who that was,*" she said, with a surprised tone in her voice.

"*Jude,*" I said without looking up.

"*How did you know?*" she asked, with true astonishment in her voice.

"*Are you kidding?*" I answered, still not looking up, "*I'm surprised he took this long to call. I'll bet he just woke up. He was probably up past four a.m. telling his drummer friend all about the French photographer he just met. So, what did he want?*"

Victorine didn't answer.

"*What did he want?*" I asked again, now looking up.

"*No . . . you really think so?*" She asked sitting down across from me.

"*What. Did. He. Want?*" I repeated, slamming my book shut.

After a long pause she answered.

"*He's coming over tomorrow. He said he wants to see the photographs I took for our stories.*"

"*I'm sure he does but he really just wants to see YOU, you idiot,*" I said.

Victorine jumped up, ran out of the room, then returned moments later and stood in front of me.

"*You're nuts. Look at me,*" she said gesturing with her hands, "*I look disgusting . . . like a fat cow.*"

"*Not at all,*" I said, "*you looked like a fat cow a few weeks ago but you look much better now that you're back to being a vegetarian.*"

"*Ouf, you're no help,*" she moaned, running out of the room.

Victorine spent the rest of the afternoon running around cleaning and straightening up our small apartment. The hum of the vacuum and the smell of cleaning agents filled the air. I noticed it was getting dark outside when she suddenly flew past me in her hat and coat and disappeared out the front door. I didn't bother to call after her to ask where she was going but instead took advantage of the quiet lull to concentrate on my studies. I had enough to worry about on my own. My first interview at the UN was in a few days and according to my friend who had helped arrange it, I would be taking a series of written and oral tests to evaluate my translation skills. I was applying for a post as a verbatim translator, reviewing the daily transcripts of the Security Council and checking them for mistakes. Accuracy was essential. Residual anxiety from my last round of failed written exams remained and frankly I was nervous. I was taking a break, making myself a cup of tea when Victorine burst in the door, arms full of grocery bags. She had been gone over two hours.

"*What's all this?*" I asked.

"*He's coming tomorrow for breakfast,*" she answered.

"*Breakfast?*"

"*Well, actually he said, 'brunch' . . . around noon.*"

She quickly unpacked her shopping bags and I could see that she had gone out to pick up some special groceries for tomorrow's "brunch": a dozen eggs, a package of flour, a package of Président butter, a carton of milk, a bag of freshly ground Columbian coffee from the gourmet shop a block past our subway station, and a simple glass vase for a bouquet of tulips which she carefully arranged and placed on the table. She stepped back, took a moment to admire her handiwork, then disappeared into the bedroom. I went back to my studying and a short time later she returned and stood in the doorway.

"Well?" she asked.

Victorine had changed into a tight black skirt and one of her nicest pink blouses. Like it or not, I was now enlisted into helping her with one last task: choosing an outfit for tomorrow.

"Too dressy for a Sunday morning," I said, shaking my head.

"Yes, you're right," she nodded, returning to the bedroom.

Realizing that any attempt at uninterrupted study was futile, I closed my book, leaned back to sip my tea and wait to see what ensemble she would come up with next. She reappeared wearing her brown corduroy jeans and heavy gray wool turtleneck sweater with red horizontal stripes.

"Are you planning to go Elk hunting?" I asked, trying not to laugh.

"Ouf," she huffed, stomping back into the bedroom.

"Oh the little liar," I sang,

"She's falling in love

Oh the little liar,

She's falling in love . . ."

I couldn't resist singing the little French schoolyard song that young children use to tease their older siblings when they first notice them showing an interest in the opposite sex. Victorine poked her head around the door, glared at me, then slid back into the bedroom. Honestly, I was happy for her. Nigel had been Victorine's first serious relationship and now, ten years out of the proverbial "pool," I sympathized with how awkward she must have felt dipping her toe back in.

She stepped back into the kitchen wearing her nicest jeans, which fit her perfectly, and a light blue blouse with an intricately embroidered floral pattern. It was MY blouse, my favorite blouse that I had been saving for a special occasion, but she looked lovely so I held my tongue and nodded.

"Perfect," I said.

Amaranth with kale and sautéed tofu

- 15 ounces of tofu, extra firm, sliced in ½ inch slices
- 1 cup of amaranth grain
- 2 cups of kale, chopped
- 1 medium purple onion, finely chopped
- 2 cups of water
- 4 tablespoons of coconut oil
- 6 tablespoons of olive oil
- 1 tablespoon of hemp seeds
- 1 pinch of sea salt
- 1 pinch of cayenne pepper

1. In a saucepan, add the amaranth, salt, pepper, and water. Cook over low heat for 25 to 30 minutes, stirring occasionally and cover.
2. Heat half of the olive oil over medium heat in a frying pan and sauté the onion until the onion begins to brown, about 3–4 minutes. Add the kale with a little water, cover and let it simmer for 10 minutes.
3. In a frying pan, add the rest of the olive oil and sauté the tofu until slightly brown on both sides.
4. Remove the amaranth from the heat and mix the coconut oil.
5. Serve the kale atop the amaranth with the fried tofu. Sprinkle with hemp seeds and salt and pepper.

Chocolate Macarons Covered with *Fleur de Sel de Guérande*

- 5 ounces of confectioner sugar
- 3.5 ounces almond powder
- 2 egg whites
- 2 tablespoons of unsweetened cacao
- 2 tablespoons of confectioner sugar
- ½ teapoon of *fleur del sel de Guérand*e (flower of salt of Guérande)

1. Preheat the oven to 320°F.
2. Mix confectioner sugar, cacao and almond powder to obtain a very thin powder.
3. Sift the powder mixture into a bowl.
4. Beat the egg white progressively adding the 2 tablespoons of confectioner sugar.
5. Once the egg whites are hard, mix them very carefully and slowly into the powder mixture.
6. Once the paste looks shiny, put it in a pastry bag and squeeze little rounds onto a parchment paper covered baking sheet.
7. Sprinkle the flower of salt on the rounds and let them rest for roughly 30–60 minutes.
8. A thin crust will develop on the rounds.
9. Place the rounds in the oven for 10–15 minutes.
10. Remove and allow to cool completely.
11. Assemble macarons by spreading the ganache on the flat side of a round and closing with another round.

The Ganache

- 10 ounces heavy cream
- 9 ounces of "grand cru" dark chocolate (such as Valrhona or Lindt
- 2 ounces of unsalted butter

1. In a saucepan bring the heavy cream to a slow boil.
2. Add the chocolate to the heavy cream, whisking it well.
3. Add butter once temperature reaches 105°F or 40°C and continue to whisk well.
4. Put the ganache in the refrigerator a couple of hours before garnishing the macarons.

A few tips: The egg white will hold better if the eggs are at room temperature. Adding a pinch of salt to the egg white will also help. All ovens are not built the same and temperature will vary. You may need two or three trials before reaching success.

Far Breton aux Pruneaux
(Baked Flan with Rum-Soaked Prunes from Brittany)
Serves 8

- 2 cups pitted prunes
- 3 tablespoons rum
- 2 tablespoons of butter to grease the pan
- 1 cup of flour
- 1 pinch of salt
- ½ cup of sugar
- 7 tablespoons of butter, melted
- 3 cups of whole milk
- 4 eggs

1. Place the pitted prunes in a bowl, add the rum, and let them sit until the prunes absorb the liquid.
2. Grease a 10-inch baking pan with butter, then pour in and evenly arrange the prunes with the leftover rum at the bottom of the baking pan.
3. In a bowl mix the flour, sugar, and salt.
4. Make a well in the center and add one by one the eggs with butter and the milk.
5. Stir it well until the batter becomes totally homogenous.
6. Pour batter on top of the prunes.
7. Bake at 350°F for 30 to 40 minutes.
8. Serve warm or cold in the baking pan.

Chapter Thirteen

From Hot Dogs to Croissants

When I awoke the next morning the apartment was filled with a delicious unmistakable sent. Victorine had gotten up early to prepare one of Maman's special dishes, *Far Breton aux Pruneaux*, baked flan with rum-soaked prunes. Whenever Maman made this at home she would prepare two dishes, place one out on the counter to cool, then hide the other high up in the cupboard out of sight.

"The mouse will soon come nibbling and this will disappear before we know it," she would whisper and wink as we giggled and promised to keep her secret.

The "mouse" to which she was referring was actually Papa who couldn't resist this tasty treat. As soon as Maman left her kitchen to attend to other housework, he would sneak in, cut himself a large slice, and gobble it up before it even had a chance to cool. Many times we caught him tiptoeing out of the kitchen licking his fingers and we would giggle again knowing we were in on both sides of our parents' secret little game. Something told me this would be the first of many *Far Breton aux Pruneaux* Victorine would make for Jude.

Victorine was setting the table when Jude rang our downstairs bell at exactly noon. I buzzed him in, opened our door, and waited on the landing as I watched him walk up the flight of stairs carrying two large white paper bags. He greeted us with a kiss on both cheeks then handed us each a bag as he entered the kitchen.

"What's this?" asked Victorine, peeking inside hers.

"I was hoping the two of you can help settle an argument," he said with a mischievous smile as he took off his coat and gloves. We both looked at him quizzically.

"My friend and I constantly argue over who makes the best croissants in Manhattan. We've narrowed it down to two places. He likes Patisserie Claude in the West Village and I prefer Ceci-Cela on Spring Street, so, I stopped by both shops this morning and picked up a half dozen from each. What do you say we turn our brunch into a croissant smack-down and settle this once and for all."

"Smack-down?" I asked.

Jude nodded and smiled excitedly.

Victorine and I looked at each other and laughed.

"And I suppose being French means we have the final say?" Victorine asked.

"I bow to your discerning palates," he replied with a mock gallant sweep of his hand.

I seriously doubted this croissant connoisseur friend of his truly existed and guessed he was having a bit of fun as an excuse to bring over far too many croissants but I played along. Then, he turned, noticed that the table already set with food and apologized for not realizing that of course, we probably had prepared something.

"Oh, no, no, no," said Victorine, "It's nothing. Croissants will be perfect."

"Okay good," said Jude, "then let's get started."

Victorine quickly cleared away her special dish, began preparing the coffee and I placed the two bags of competing croissants on the table.

It's true, croissants always taste best fresh and *Far Breton aux Pruneaux* tastes best when it's allowed to sit and the flavor of the rum soaked prunes seeps into the flan.

"Mind if I use your bathroom?" asked Jude, "I'd like to wash my hands."

"Of course, right through there," said Victorine pointing the way.

When he was safely out of earshot with the bathroom closed and water running in the sink I whispered to Victorine.

"He's adorable. Smart and silly at the same time."

Victorine just nodded with a mischievous smile as she poured boiling water into the coffee press. Then she opened the kitchen closet, rummaged inside her camera bag, pulled out her notebook and pencil, and placed them on the table next to her seat. I could tell she was ready to have a little fun. Jude returned and we all sat down at the table to begin.

"Where is this bag from?" asked Victorine as she removed three croissants from the first bag and carefully placed one on each of our plates.

"That one's from Patisserie Claude," answered Jude.

Victorine opened her notebook and wrote "PC" at the top of a blank page.

"Now," she said, "Watch and learn how an expert judges a croissant. First, the crust. We start by judging the crust with our eyes."

Jude and I looked at each other and giggled.

"The ideal crust should have an even, golden brown color on the entire surface," she said as she carefully examined her croissant, "Hmm, I give this one an eight point five."

She wrote her score in her notebook as we in turn examined our own crusts.

"Next, the crust should be distinct from the interior. It should be very flaky and shatter or crumble when you tear it," she said.

She then picked up her croissant with her left hand, pinched a piece of the end with her right hand and slowly tore it off.

"Not bad," she said, noting a few small crumbs of crust that had fallen on her plate.

Jude and I followed suit, fighting back our urge to laugh.

"Now, it's time for the tongue test," she continued, "each layer of the crust should almost melt on your tongue but not feel greasy on your hands."

She popped the end piece into her mouth and closed her eyes. She opened them after a moment then rubbed her thumb and fingers together.

"Hmm, crisp, not greasy . . . not bad," she said with a nod, "I give that another eight point five."

She made a few scribbles in her notebook.

"So, that's a total score of seventeen for the crust. Next, the interior."

"What?" asked Jude. "All that just for the crust?"

Victorine leaned back in her chair, arched her eyebrow, and gave him a withering look.

"I thought you took your croissants seriously," she said totally straight faced, "let me know now if I'm just wasting my time because I can just as well . . ."

"No, no, no," he said apologetically, "please go on."

I fought hard to keep a straight face. Poor Jude, he had no idea what he was getting himself into. Victorine paused before she continued.

"Okay," she said finally, "Now, the interior should have many layers and they should all be feathery-light, moist but not gummy or doughy . . ."

She pulled another section away from the croissant.

" . . . and each layer should have some stretch as you pull it away with your fingers but they should still separate gently."

She popped the next piece in her mouth as Jude and I pulled apart our own croissants and judged the stretchiness.

"Hmm," she said raising her eyebrows and nodding her head, "again, not bad. Not bad at all. I give the interior a nine."

She jotted down her score in her notebook and added a few numbers.

"Okay, we're up to a total of twenty-six for crust and interior, but now . . ." she said solemnly holding up her finger, " . . . the most important factor . . . flavor. This score is most important and it counts double."

Jude listened intently. He was hanging on her every word. Victorine was incredible. I had no idea where she was coming up with this stuff but she was on a roll.

"Now," she continued, "the flavor of the perfect croissant should be intensely buttery and the sweetness should come from the natural sweetness of dairy. It shouldn't taste as if there was added sugar and it should be well-seasoned but not so salty so you couldn't imagine eating it with a little jam or preserves."

With that she popped the remainder in her mouth and took a long moment to savor its flavor. She slowly opened her eyes and gave a nod of approval.

"For flavor, she said, "this gets . . ."

Jude leaned forward and sat wide-eyed, waiting for the verdict.

" . . . an eight point five."

She scribbled her calculations in her notebook.

"Let's see . . . times two . . . Wow, that's a total of forty-three," she said nodding as if impressed.

I couldn't resist joining in on her little game.

"Really?" I exclaimed, "That's one of the highest scores yet."

Victorine removed three croissants from the second bag and placed one on each of our plates. She then put her notebook down in front of Jude.

"Okay," she said, "now it's your turn. Let's see how your croissants from Ceci-Cela rate."

We went through the entire excruciating process again, helping Jude painstakingly dissect and rate his croissant. Unfortunately, once tallied, its score only added up to thirty-nine.

"Oh, no," I sighed, "It looks as if your friend was right. The croissants from Patisserie Claude are better."

"Well," he said sheepishly, "actually, I was just teasing."

"About what?" asked Victorine.

"About my friend and I having an argument," he answered, "I just made up that story so you wouldn't think I was crazy for bringing over so many croissants."

We cleared the dishes and I while made some fresh coffee Victorine got her photo portfolio from the closet and spread it out on the table. Jude carefully examined each print that we had submitted with our articles and listened intently as we told him details of our adventures. He insisted on examining all the tiny photos on the contact sheets that hadn't been blown up into full-size prints. As he sat hunched over the table, peering through the loupe, Victorine caught my eye and I gave her an approving nod.

"You know," he said, "I was thinking last night about all the stories you told me and now that I've seen these photos I'm convinced. You should write a book about your adventures."

"But we already wrote the articles," I said with a shrug.

"I know," he said, "but they're in French. What I'm suggesting is you write it in English . . . for the American audience. Trust me, you two have seen a side of America that most Americans know nothing about . . . have never seen. Not only that, as Europeans you have a unique perspective. Seriously, include some of these amazing photographs and you've got something really special."

He looked at us both, nodded his head slowly and assuredly then went back to examining the contact sheets through the loupe. I didn't give his suggestion much thought, excused myself saying I had some studying to do and went to the bedroom to read. I could hear them talking softly, occasionally laughing and about an hour or so later Victorine came into the bedroom to get her coat.

"We're going to go out to hear a friend of his who's playing downtown. Do you mind?" she asked.

"Don't be silly," I said.

"Do you want to come?" she asked.

"Get out of here," I said as I threw a pillow at her.

"Don't wait up."

"I won't."

"Goodbye Natasha," Jude called from the kitchen.

"Goodbye Jude. Thank you for the croissants."

I heard the front door shut and their footsteps fade as they descended the stairs. Later, when I took a break from studying and went to the kitchen to make a cup of tea, I discovered that two little mice had eaten half of the *Far Breton aux Pruneaux.*

If I had to pick a day, I would say that Sunday marked the close of our first chapter in America. I passed all my exams at the UN the following week and officially started my new job three weeks later. It was a difficult post, with long hours and insane deadlines but the fast pace and interaction with an eclectic group of interesting people made it very rewarding. Victorine found a job as a camera operator at a TV station, then left to work as a tour guide, then a chef, then . . . I lost track. That was Victorine. She thrived on new experiences. What did stay consistent for her though was Jude. They fell head over heels in love and became inseparable. Eventually she moved out of our apartment and into a house upstate with Jude. It wasn't quite a farm but it was a place out of the city with a yard big enough for a large vegetable garden. It turned out that he also longed to live in the countryside.

The last time we all got together was when our cousin Roger came to visit from France. He stayed at my apartment and Victorine and Jude drove into Manhattan to join us for a whirlwind tour of the city. It was a perfect beautiful sunny spring day and we brought him to all the tourist sites: the Empire State Building, Times Square, Greenwich Village, and South Street Seaport where we found a little seafood restaurant to stop for lunch. I ordered their specialty, Manhattan Clam Chowder and the first spoonful brought me back to the wonderful *soupe aux poissons* or fish soup we would get at our favorite restaurant in Concarneau, the beautiful walled seaside town near our home in Brittany. Sitting at the table with Victorine, Jude, and Roger, I felt a twinge of nostalgia mixed with the anticipation one feels when poised at the edge of life's next chapter.

We ended the day with a ferry ride out to visit Lady Liberty. Victorine and I hadn't seen her since our first day in America and as we walked around the island, gazing up from below, we once again burst into song, "I'm singing with you, liberty!" The sun, close to setting, was beginning to glow red when we boarded the last ferry back to Manhattan. I turned for one last look and saw Lady Liberty looking down at me and smiling.

Manhattan Clam Chowder
Serves 6

- 1 cup of baby clams
- 3 cups of clam broth
- 2 cups can diced tomatoes
- 1 cup chopped onion
- 2 potatoes, peeled and chopped in small cubes
- ½ cup finely chopped carrots
- 2 garlic cloves, finely chopped
- ¼ cup of fresh parsley, chopped
- 2 dried bay leaves
- 2 teaspoons dried oregano
- Salt and freshly ground pepper to taste

1. In a large saucepan pour clam broth, tomatoes, onions, potatoes, carrots, garlic, thyme, oregano, bay leaves, salt, freshly ground pepper, and thyme.
2. Cover and cook on low heat for 35 to 40 minutes.
3. Remove the pan from the heat.
4. Mash the vegetables slightly to thicken the broth.
5. Add clams to the saucepan and heat thoroughly for 10 minutes.
6. Pour soup in bowls, sprinkle fresh parsley, and serve hot.

Leabharlanna Poibli Chathair Bhaile Átha Cliath
Dublin City Public Libraries